Physical Education for Learning

Also available from Continuum

Getting the Buggers Fit 2nd Edition, Lorraine Cale and Joanne Harris
Teaching Physical Education 11–18, Tony Macfadyen and Richard Bailey
Teaching Physical Education in the Primary School, Ian Pickup and Lawry Price

Physical Education for Learning
A Guide for Secondary Schools

Edited by

Richard Bailey

Resources to accompany this book are available online at: www.richardbailey.net

Please visit the link and register with us to receive your password and to access these downloadable resources.

If you experience any problems accessing the resources, please contact Continuum at: info@continuumbooks.com

continuum

Continuum International Publishing Group

The Tower Building   80 Maiden Lane
11 York Road   Suite 704
London, SE1 7NX   New York, NY 10038

www.continuumbooks.com

British Library Cataloguing-in-Publication Data
A catalogue record for this book is available from the British Library.
ISBN: 9781847065025 (paperback)

Library of Congress Cataloging-in-Publication Data
Physical education for learning: a guide for secondary schools/edited by Richard Bailey.
    p. cm.
ISBN: 978-1-84706-502-5 (pbk.)
1. Physical education and training–Study and teaching (Secondary)–Great Britain.
2. Physical education teachers–Training of–Great Britain. I. Bailey, Richard, 1966-
II. Title.

GV365.5.G7P49 2010
613.7'0430941–dc22   2009030757

Typeset by Newgen Imaging Systems Pvt Ltd, Chennai, India
Printed and bound in Great Britain by the MPG Books Group

Contents

Foreword

The main criteria used by the afPE (Association for Physical Education) for quality physical education are a focus on learning, and inclusion, that is, that programmes of delivery meet the needs of every child, whatever their learning needs or interests. It is therefore heartening to be writing a Foreword to a physical education book, whose focus is squarely on physical education for learning. The recurrent themes of differentiation and progression as keys to quality learning are welcome, as is the expectation that readers of the book are themselves being expected to become active and reflective learners. The range and quality of contributions are impressive, from leaders in the profession with genuine experience and informed reflection. They may use different lenses, but the focus is always on the processes and outcomes of learning. The contributors also reflect and celebrate the history and culture of physical education's development, as well as highlighting the need for practice and research to inform each other.

I enjoy Richard Bailey's challenge in the Preface, about the outcomes of teaching, too often taken for granted as effective learning. Of course, it is not easy to demonstrate that learning has taken place: it cannot be seen or touched, and evidence of learning has to be inferred from observed behaviour. But it is all too easy to identify when learning has been less than accurate or effective. I well remember leading a course of study on the early years of national leisure surveys, during which I tried very hard to expose the limitations and flaws of national surveys, especially for identifying or understanding causal relationships. I must have tried too hard, as I learned when I read one of my students' view – 'the largely useless national recreation surveys'!

Learning is problematic, and in physical education, success and failure are very public. The various contributors to this reader have recognized this, and provided outlines of issues and challenges which, used well, should support physical education teachers' pride in their endeavours to help children and young people learn and enjoy the skills, knowledge and understanding which characterize physical education.

It is good to see questioned, the dominance of the sport model, and its influence on physical education, especially in secondary schools and specialist sports colleges. This emphasizes that physical education, as all other 'subjects' is socially constructed and subject to change through influence and political direction. There are several insightful glances at the limitations of infrastructure, strategies and government rhetoric and expectation, redirecting attention to the everyday, ever-increasing demands on secondary specialist teachers of physical education.

Hence, the various contributors illuminate the notions of professionalism and professional communities in teaching, and the fact that teachers matter. Their experience and skills, interacting with learners' voices and encounters, constitute the basis of the challenge and review which is essential for effective learning. They also show the breadth and wealth of physical education's learning experiences and contexts, providing a rich variety of ways of knowing and developing. The coverage of issues is itself a framework for the integrity and distinctive nature of physical education, and the joys and challenges of leading and guiding learners, within this unmatchable environment of movement, physical engagement and endeavour, individual and group efforts and achievements.

Margaret Talbot

Professor Margaret Talbot, PhD OBE FRSA
Chief Executive, Association for Physical Education

Preface

The one-time English Secretary of State for Education Kenneth Clarke is reported to have said 'having any ideas about how children learn, or develop, or feel, should be seen as a subversive activity'. Apparently, his statement was prompted by his frustration with teachers who wilfully discussed questions like 'how do children learn?' and 'how can we support this learning?' Implicit in Clarke's statement is a common view that learning is a simple matter. In many cases, the assumption is that teaching *becomes* learning: I teach, you learn; if I teach and you don't learn, it must be your fault! A moment's reflection will show that this is utter nonsense.

Have you ever been taught a subject that made no sense to you? Or have you managed to recall just enough to say the right words in response to a question, but that you recognized you really did not understand, and certainly wouldn't be able to apply? Have you ever sat patiently while someone tried to teach you something that was of no interest to you? Have you ever cursed your inability to make some skill or knowledge 'stick'? Have you ever thought you had learned something, but you immediately forgot it a moment later? Of course you have. We have all had these sorts of experiences, which can be frustrating for the learner, and disappointing for the teacher. It happens all of the time, because learning is complex. This is one reason why secondary physical education needs to be taught by qualified professionals rather than the 'keen mums and dads' occasionally promoted by simple-minded politicians. It is not difficult to set up a game of football among a small group of enthusiastic children. It is more difficult to motivate and engage a large and diverse group of young people so that each leaves the session not just having been occupied, but also having learned something valuable, inspired for future physical activity.

The fundamental responsibility of teachers is to promote learning. All other roles – management, administration, policing, pastoral care – are secondary to learning. Indeed, these additional roles are mainly justified in terms of their ability to support learning. This is all too easy to forget in physical education where the observer might consider a lesson a success when the pupils are 'busy, happy and good', irrespective of whether or not they are learning anything. As superficially attractive as this conception of 'good PE' might at first seem, it needs to be rejected as it barely qualifies for a physical *education* at all. Rather, it is an expensively supervised break time. Physical education, if that term is to have any meaning, requires a focus on pupils' learning.

With this in mind, the book that you are holding in your hands has a clear and explicit focus – PHYSICAL EDUCATION FOR LEARNING. The chapters – written by some of the leading writers and teachers of physical education – discuss ways in which physical activities can be planned, presented, organized and assessed in support of learning.

Each chapter introduces and develops the central ideas and principles of effective practice. You will find numerous opportunities to reflect on your own experiences. Please take these directed tasks seriously and invest time in working through the activities as they will contribute enormously to your own learning. You will also find suggestions for further reading and study, labelled 'Learning More'. These books are important and will more than repay your investment in coming to terms with the ideas they explore.

Physical education can and does have a transformational effect on young people. It is the only subject of the timetable specifically concerned with physical skills and bodies. As such, it is intimately connected with young people's conceptions about themselves as learners and as human beings. Physical education teachers matter. We sincerely hope that this book helps you to become a teacher who really makes a difference to young people's lives. It is well worth the effort!

The Editor

Richard Bailey is a writer and theorist on physical education, sport and education. A former teacher, he has been a Professor at Canterbury, Roehampton and most recently Birmingham Universities. He has studied Physical Education, Philosophy and Anthropology, and continues to work in these areas, especially with regard to their relevance for learning and the development of expertise. Dr Bailey has undertaken funded research in every continent of the world. He works with UNESCO as Expert Adviser, the World Health Organisation, the European Union, and many similar agencies. He has carried out work on behalf of the English, Scottish and Welsh governments, numerous educational and sports agencies. Dr Bailey was Director of the most comprehensive review ever published on the Benefits of Physical Education and Sport (2007–2008), Co-director of the UK's independent review of player development in sport (2008–2009), and advisor for the Agency for Cooperation in Secondary Education in post-conflict societies (2006–2008). In 2004 he was selected by delegates from more than 200 countries to act as Rapporteur for UNESCO's Athens Declaration. He is the author of more than 100 research papers, articles and reports, and has written or co-written 15 books on educational topics. His recent books include *Handbook of Philosophy of Education* (Sage, with Robin Barrow, David Carr and McCarthy, 2009), *Long-term Engagement in Sport* (ICSSPE, with Nicholas Holt, 2009), *The Routledge Physical Education Reader* (with David Kirk, 2009), *Meeting the Needs of Your Most Able Pupils* (David Fulton, with David Morley, 2008). His website is www.richardbailey.net; and weblog is Talking Education and Sport (http://talkingeducationandsport.blogspot.com/).

The Contributors

Kathleen Armour is Professor of Physical Education and Sport Pedagogy, and Director of Research, in the School of Sport, Exercise and Health Sciences at Loughborough University, UK. Her research interests centre on professional development for teachers and coaches. In particular, Professor Armour is interested in effective, career-long professional development for teachers and coaches, and in PE teachers' learning needs in the areas of health and vulnerable children.

Lorraine Cale is a senior lecturer in the School of Sport and Exercise Sciences at Loughborough University and is Director of the PGCE Physical Education Teacher Education (PETE) programme. Her teaching and research lie in the areas of Physical Education, PETE, and physical activity promotion in young people, both within and beyond the curriculum. Lorraine has been involved in training teachers and designing and delivering continuing professional development courses for teachers for many years. She has also presented at numerous national and international conferences and published her work in academic and professional journals.

Fiona C. Chambers joined the Department of Education at University College Cork, Ireland, in 2006. Having taught Physical Education for 11 years at Secondary Level, Fiona currently lectures in the pedagogy of Sport and PE. Fiona's research interests centre on effective teacher professional learning across the career span, with a particular focus on Initial Teacher Education. Her PhD, awarded in 2008, focused on student teacher learning during teaching practice. Most recently, Fiona has been funded by the Teaching Council in Ireland to examine the role of mentoring in Teaching Practice as a PE student teacher learning tool.

Suzanne Everley graduated from the University of Warwick and taught in Japan prior to returning to university to complete an MA in Sport, Culture and Society. She taught in Further Education for five years before completing her PhD in 'Children's Experiences of Physical Education'. Suzanne became a senior lecturer in Initial Teacher Training in physical education at the University of Chichester in 2002. Her main role focuses on the teaching of sociological issues within physical education and sport at undergraduate and post-graduate levels. Suzanne has a continued research interest in the experiences of young people and physical education/physical activity.

Rebecca Duncombe has worked as a Research Associate in the Institute of Youth Sport at Loughborough University, UK, since March 2005. Her PhD focused on primary school teachers and their professional learning in physical education. Rebecca has been primarily engaged in research on national projects that use sport and physical activity as a 'vehicle' that can re-engage disaffected young people in education (e.g. BSkyB/YST 'Living for Sport' and Deutsche Bank 'Moving Generations'). Prior to joining the university, Rebecca was employed as a primary school teacher with responsibility for co-ordinating PE.

Andrew Frapwell was a teacher for ten years, before taking up an appointment at the University of Worcester in Initial Teacher Training for eight years, where he was a principal lecturer and curriculum leader for physical education, also leading the PGCE Secondary Physical Education Course. Andrew now works as an Independent Education Consultant, and is currently the afPE and CfBT Education Trust National Subject Lead for physical education responsible for the dissemination and implementation support for the new secondary curriculum in England. He has nationally led work on Assessment for learning for afPE and QCA producing many resources and web-based materials for educators. This focus is linked to his research which has been presented in the UK, USA, Europe and New Zealand.

Enrique García Bengoechea is an assistant professor in the Department of Kinesiology and Physical Education at McGill University in Canada, where he teaches courses in health and lifestyle education and physical education curriculum development. Enrique is interested in the study of youth sport and physical education programs as developmental interventions and health promotion opportunities.

Jo Harris has 12 years experience of teaching physical education in schools and 20 years experience in higher education. She is a senior lecturer in physical education and Director of the Teacher Education Unit at Loughborough University. Her research focuses on the expression of health within school physical education. Jo has produced numerous teaching resources and delivered many professional development courses. She has presented at national and international conferences and has published in professional and academic journals. Jo was President of the Physical Education Association of the United Kingdom and is currently Deputy Chair of the Association for Physical Education.

Carmel Hinchion is a lecturer in Teaching, Learning and Assessment at the University of Limerick (UL). She works with initial teacher education undergraduate and post-graduate students and on the Counselling and Guidance programme for qualified teachers. Her research interests include the developing identities of student teachers, English pedagogy, the arts in education, reflective practice and counselling theory and practice.

Gary D. Kinchin is a senior lecturer in physical education at the University of Southampton, England. He has held a number of positions of responsibility within the School of Education, most recently serving as Deputy Head of School. Gary completed his MA and PhD at The Ohio State University and has held academic appointments at De Montfort University and Illinois State University. His research interests focus on Sport Education and on physical education teacher education. Gary is a member of the editorial board of *Physical Education and Sport Pedagogy* and PE ITTE Network Advisory Board.

David Kirk has published widely on physical education and youth sport. He was Dean of the Carnegie Faculty of Sport and Education at Leeds Metropolitan University between 2005–2008, and is currently the Alexander Chair of Sport and Physical Education at the University of Bedfordshire. He is founding editor of the Routledge journal *Physical Education and Sport Pedagogy*.

Matthew Light has 13 years experience of working in secondary schools and 5 years working in initial teacher education. He is a senior lecturer in physical education at Canterbury Christ Church University, England. His research interests include the use of ICT in physical education and psychological constructs in physical education. Matthew has worked with colleagues on national research projects and is involved with international teaching institutions in the delivery of teacher education in South East Asia.

Rebecca J. Lloyd is an assistant professor in Faculty of Education at the University of Ottawa in Canada who promotes inter-disciplinarity in health and physical education by combining principles of pedagogy, sport psychology and curriculum understanding. In collaboration with Stephen Smith, she has developed a motion-sensitive phenomenological approach to research and has explored the experience of flow in exercise pedagogy and the presence of vitality in physical education. Currently, Stephen and Rebecca are developing a 'Physical Mindfulness Model' that fleshes out kinaesthetic pathways towards experiencing enhanced flow and vitality in physical education, physical activity and sport performance contexts.

Tony Macfadyen is Senior Lecturer in Education at the University of Reading where he is Head of Physical Education. He is also the Programme Leader for PGCE and GTP Secondary Physical Education courses and is the author of two influential Physical Education books (with Richard Bailey). His research interests focus upon teaching styles, lesson structure and student–mentor lesson observation discussions. Previously he taught physical education both in England and internationally and was Head of Physical Education at the Garden International School, Malaysia. Currently he is Vice Chair of AfPE (South East) and a member of the BERA Special Interest Group for Physical Education and Sport Pedagogy.

Ann MacPhail is Senior Lecturer in the Department of Physical Education and Sport Sciences at UL, Ireland. Prior to joining the faculty at UL Ann was a Research Associate at Loughborough University. Ann has a B.Ed (Honours) Physical Education Degree from Heriot Watt University, Edinburgh and a PhD from the University of Glasgow. Ann's main teaching and research interests revolve around physical education teacher education, young people in sport, curriculum development in physical education, teaching, learning and assessment issues within school physical education, methodological issues in working with young people and ethnography. Ann is Associate Editor for Physical Education and Sport Pedagogy and is co-editing a book on young people's voices in physical education and youth sport with Mary O'Sullivan.

Kyriaki Makopoulou was appointed as a lecturer in the School of Education at the University of Birmingham, UK, in September 2008. Kyriaki has an undergraduate degree from the University of Athens, and an MSc in Physical Education (with Distinction) from Loughborough University. Her PhD (awarded in 2009) focused on the nature of PE teachers' engagement in career-long professional learning and its impact upon practice, and this is her current research focus. Between 20005 and 2008 Kyriaki, together with Professor Armour, undertook an independent evaluation of the National Continuing Professional Development Programme for PE teachers in England.

David Morley has been involved in multi-skills development for the past six years. During his time at Leeds Metropolitan University, within his role as Director of the Research Unit in Talent Development in PE and Sport, he established Carnegie Multi-skills Talent Camps involving children from across Yorkshire. He continues to act as an advisor to the Youth Sport Trust and has been instrumental in the development of national talent development and multi-skills strategies. He has published extensively in these areas, developed resources, delivered CPD for coaches and teachers and presented his work at national and international conferences. His latest involvement in nurturing children's movement competencies is in developing multi-skills on the school playground, and he heads a national initiative with Education and Special Projects (ESP).

Mary O'Sullivan is currently Dean of the Faculty of Education and Health Sciences and Co-Director of the Physical Education, Physical Activity and Youth Sport (PE PAYS) Research Centre at UL. Her teaching and research interests focus on the preparation of new teachers, professional development for experienced teachers, and quality physical education and sport experiences for young people. She is keen to influence policy research and development in support of high quality teaching and access for all young people to fun and meaningful physical activity cultures.

Graham Parton is a principal lecturer in Professional Studies at Leeds Metropolitan University. Before starting this role in January 2009, he was a senior lecturer at Canterbury Christ Church University where he led the second year of the BA (Hons) in Primary Education. Graham's research interests include student learning in professional education and creativity in ICT education. Graham is currently completing his PhD in the area of student experience while engaging in a problem-based learning curriculum and has published and presented this research at a number of conferences.

Lesley Phillpots is a lecturer in the School of Education at the University of Birmingham. She is Programme Leader for a BA in Sport, Physical Education and Coaching Science and also delivers on post-graduate teacher education courses in secondary and primary physical education within the College of Social Sciences. Prior to joining the University of Birmingham, Lesley trained as a secondary PE teacher and taught in both secondary and primary schools in the UK. Her research focuses on government policy for sport and school sport and in particular the work of specialist sports colleges, school sport partnerships and national governing bodies of sport in the UK.

Stephen J. Smith is Associate Professor and Director of Professional Programs at Simon Fraser University. His scholarly work pertains to curricular and instructional practices in physical education, health education and teacher education. Illustrative publications are the 1997 book *Risk and Our Pedagogical Relation to Children: On the Playground and Beyond*, and the 2004 book *The Bearing of Inquiry in Teacher Education*. His recent work addresses vitality and physical mindfulness as overarching concepts of physical education and, more broadly speaking, of a somatic approach to teacher education. His scholarship draws inspiration from a range of traditional and alternative movement disciplines from swimming to circus and equestrian arts.

Jon Spence is Principal Lecturer, Subject Leader and Enterprise Manager for Physical Education at Roehampton University. He has had been involved in the teaching of physical education for more than 20 years, initially as a teacher and head of department and for the last 8 years as a teacher educator. Jon was involved in the original development of 'A' Level Physical Education, as a co-author of a key 'A' Level text, and as an examination paper scrutineer.

Deborah Tannehill is a senior lecturer in the Department of Physical Education and Sport Sciences at UL. She is Course Director for the Graduate Diploma in Education – Physical Education, Course Director of the MSc in Teaching Physical Education, and Co-Director of the Physical Education, Physical Activity and Youth Sport (PE PAYS) Research Centre. Deborah has conducted research on teaching and teacher education in physical education, and publishes frequently in both scholarly and applied journals. Currently her work is focused on curriculum development, assessment and instruction. Prior to joining the faculty at UL Deborah was Professor and Assistant Dean at Pacific Lutheran University (PLU) and Professor at the Ohio State University.

Philip Vickerman is Professor of Inclusive Education and Learning in the Faculty of Education, Community and Leisure at Liverpool John Moores University. Philip works nationally and internationally on aspects of inclusive physical education and has advised governments and professional associations. Philip is a National Teaching Fellow awarded by the Higher Education Academy in recognition of his contribution to the field of inclusive education. He has written extensively in journals and books on special educational needs and is also an external examiner on an Erasmus Mundus European Masters in Adapted Physical Activity.

Peter Whitlam is the project manager for health and safety and lead tutor for risk management courses with the Association for Physical Education and is an independent consultant.

He holds higher degrees in law and physical education; is the author of *Case Law in Physical Education: A Guide to Good Practice* (2004); a contributor and co-author to five editions of *Safe Practice in Physical Education and School Sport* (BAALPE , now afPE); has contributed to other publications on risk assessment in physical education and is a trained legal expert witness. He also tutors a university course on sports law at Oxford Brookes University.

Andy Wild has worked at the University of Chichester since 2007. Previously, he worked for the afPE and prior to that he was the Continuing Professional Development Manager for the Physical Education Association for the United Kingdom (PEA UK). Andy is an active (Honoured) member of the Association for Physical Education; in 2006/07 he edited the inaugural Members Yearbook. In 2005 Andy was awarded a *Fellowship of PEA UK* in recognition of his outstanding contribution to the aims and objectives of the Association. Between 1986 and 1999 he taught and managed physical education in a large secondary school in South-East England.

List of Abbreviations and Acronyms

afPE	Association for Physical Education
AfL	Assessment for Learning
ALT	Academic Learning Time
ALT-PE	Academic Learning Time in Physical Education
BAALPE	British Association of Advisors and Lecturers in Physical Education
CPD	Continuing Professional Development
CR	Conditioned response
CS	Conditioned stimulus
DCMS	Department for Culture, Media and Sport
DCFS	Department for Children, Schools and Families
DfES	Department for Education and Skills
DoH	Department of Health
ESP	Education and Special Projects
GPS	Global Positioning System
HRE	Health-related exercise
ICSSPE	International Council of Sport Science and Physical Education
ILO	Intended Learning Outcomes
IYS	Institute of Youth Sport
LEA	Local Education Authority
NASPE	National Association of Sport and Physical Education
NCPE	National Curriculum Physical Education
NICE	National Institute for Health and Clinical Excellence
PEA UK	Physical Education Association for the United Kingdom
PESSCL	Physical Education, School Sport and Club Links
PE PAYS	Physical Education, Physical Activity and Youth Sport
PESS	Physical Education and School Sport
PETE	Physical Education Teacher Education
PLC	Professional learning community
PLU	Pacific Lutheran University
PSA	Public service agreement
QCA	Qualifications and Curriculum Authority

QTS	Qualified Teacher Status
RSS	Really Simple Syndication
SCAA	School Curriculum and Assessment Authority
SSP	School Sport Partnership
TDA	Training and Development Agency for Schools
TGfU	Teaching Games for Understanding
TLRP/ESRC	Teaching and Learning Research Programme/Economic and Social Research Council in the UK
UCR	Unconditioned response
UCS	Unconditioned stimulus
UL	University of Limerick
USDHHS	United States Department of Health and Human Services

Part One
Thinking about Physical Education

Becoming a Teacher

1

Lorraine Cale

Welcome to teaching and more specifically to physical education teaching. As a trainee or newly qualified teacher, you are embarking on a stimulating, rewarding but challenging career. Equally, the process of becoming and developing as a physical education teacher should be stimulating, rewarding and challenging. The process of learning to teach and the skills and qualities required of effective teachers are considered later in this chapter. Initially though, to become a teacher of physical education, or of any subject, commitment to both teaching and your subject are essential. First and foremost you will be a teacher of children, and will require generic knowledge, skills, and qualities to equip you to work effectively with young people. Secondly, the context within which you will spend a good deal, though not all, of your time will be physical education and therefore subject specific knowledge and skills will also be required.

In addition, you will need to understand yourself, including your values, beliefs or 'philosophies', and be able to reflect on how these influence your teaching and pupils' learning. In effect, you should aim to become an informed and reflective practitioner. To achieve this, you will need to be committed to your own learning and professional development and see this as a lifelong process which begins during your initial teacher training (ITT) and continues throughout your career. Furthermore, whilst teacher training and teaching is practical in terms of developing skills and teaching methods, it is also concerned with theory. Attention to theory, such as is covered within this text, should therefore inform your practice and influence your decisions concerning what to do as a physical education teacher and why and how to do it.

This introductory chapter aims to help you to begin to appreciate and reflect on teaching, physical education teaching, and what is involved in becoming a teacher of physical education. In this way, it should help you to more adequately prepare for and manage what lies ahead.

The Importance of Teaching and Physical Education

Just as teaching is a stimulating, rewarding and challenging career, as exemplified by the following quote, it is also a very important career and one which carries with it great responsibility:

> Teaching is the most important job in our society. Every other occupation relies on the skills, expertise and enthusiasm of teachers. (General Teaching Council, 2003)

Indeed, Armour (2006, p. 203) illustrates the potential influence teachers have when she notes how 'over a 35-year career, a single teacher could teach approximately 30,000 lessons to anything up to 100,000 pupils'. In addition, some of the publicity messages that have been employed by the Training and Development Agency for Schools (TDA) in England in recent years highlight the responsibility, yet also the rewards of teaching. Examples include:

- Make a positive difference to your own and others' lives – teach.
- You never forget a good teacher.
- Work with the most exciting people in the country – teach.

With regards to physical education teaching, it has been suggested that 'there are few subjects as important for children's development and general education as physical educa-tion . . .' and that the contribution it can make 'is both distinctive and significant' (Bailey, 2005, p. xi). The aims of physical education are explored in the next chapter, consideration of which clearly highlight its importance within the curriculum. Briefly with respect to the benefits though, physical education can have a positive effect on children's physical, lifestyle, affective, social and cognitive development (Bailey, 2009).

Reflection

First, to encourage you to begin to fully appreciate and reflect on the importance of teaching, physical education teaching, becoming a physical education teacher, and what these involve, consider the questions below. How much prior attention have you paid to these? If possible, discuss your ideas and responses with another trainee or newly qualified teacher. Some of these questions and/or the issues raised by these will be addressed later within this or subsequent chapters.

- What is teaching?
- What is physical education? What are its aims?
- What is a physically educated person?
- Why do I want to teach and teach physical education specifically?
- What do I wish to achieve as a physical education teacher?
- What are my beliefs, values and philosophies concerning education and physical education? How have these been formed?

Reasons for Becoming a Physical Education Teacher

Studies on teacher recruitment and retention have consistently revealed that trainee teachers are attracted to the profession largely for intrinsic reasons related to the profession itself, a desire to continue with the subject and personal fulfilment, and due to the positive experiences they had while they were at school (Edmonds et al., 2002; Younger et al., 2004). The reasons people give for wanting to become a physical education teacher largely concur with these and centre around an enjoyment or love of sport and/or physical education; the positive influences of their own physical education teachers; their own ability and success in sport and/or physical education; a desire to pass on their knowledge, enthusiasm and love to others; and a desire to work with young people (Evans and Williams, 1989; Mawer, 1995; Capel, 2005a).

Reflection

Compare the above reasons for wanting to teach with your own from the previous activity.

1. To what extent do these reasons reflect you own?
2. Why do you think this is?

Whilst the above might reflect your own and seem valid reasons for wanting to teach physical education, as is noted in the next section, such reasons and the values, attitudes and beliefs underlying them may raise issues. Also, one of these reasons on its own may not be adequate. Ideally a desire to teach should be rooted within one's subject as well as within a desire to work with young people.

Physical Education Teachers' Philosophies

Much has been written about physical education teachers' values and beliefs (e.g. Kirk, 1992; Green, 2003, 2009; Tsangaridou, 2006), or in other words their 'philosophies', and consistencies in their philosophies have been found. Whilst many physical education teachers' philosophies incorporate several ideas or ideologies regarding the nature and purpose of physical education, the most prominent theme is that of sport (Green, 2009). Other key themes include: health, academic value, education for leisure, sport (participation) for all, and enjoyment (Kirk, 1992; Green, 2003, 2009). However, even when teachers cite other aspects such as health or participation as important, sport (and often competitive sport and team games), is still seen as the main vehicle for achieving these. Furthermore, it has been noted how physical education teachers' philosophies tend to reflect their prior physical education experiences and sporting practice suggesting that they tend to hold traditional views and beliefs of their subject (Green, 2009). Indeed, such a traditional view of physical education teachers is not uncommon.

The above is significant in that teachers' values, attitudes and beliefs influence their practice. Thus, given that many young people do not enjoy or achieve success in sport, the dominance of a sporting ideology is likely to present challenges and even frustrations for teachers and pupils alike. It is therefore important to be aware of your own philosophies and reflect on how they might influence your teaching. In addition, you need to consider how you might deal with and engage pupils in your classes with differing values, attitudes and beliefs from your own.

Effective Teaching

Most people would agree with the TDA publicity message 'You never forget a good teacher' and you can probably recall a favourite teacher from our own school days who you perhaps aspire to be like. However, what made them 'good'?

Reflection

Make a list of the skills and qualities you feel are required of a 'good' teacher. Then, read the following section and compare your list with the skills and qualities identified in the text. Note the similarities and differences.

Good teachers are considered to be effective teachers and research on teacher effectiveness provides an insight into the skills and qualities required and the processes by which teachers become effective. Siedentop and Tannehill (2000) draw the analogy between learning to teach effectively and learning to be good at sport. They state:

> If you want to get better, you have to know a lot about the skills and strategies of the sport, practice frequently under good conditions, and get help in the form of instruction, supervision and feedback from those who know more than you do. (p. 3)

Further, they go onto say that once those skills are gained, sufficient motivation to continually maintain and improve them is required. Related to this is that a good teacher also regularly reflects upon his or her practice (Behets and Vergauwen, 2006). Thus, in the first instance to become an effective teacher requires continued hard work, commitment, motivation, practice and reflection, supported by clear guidance and quality feedback.

The general picture that emerges of an effective teacher within the literature is of a teacher who believes he or she can make a difference, develops a management system that helps pupils stay on task, plans and implements an action-oriented programme, motivates pupils, and holds them accountable yet within a supportive and respectful climate (Siedentop and Tannehill, 2000). Siedentop and Tannehill (2000) refer to this type of teacher as the 'active teacher' who keeps students consistently engaged, uses different instructional approaches, supervises work carefully, and who consequently establishes classes where pupils are seldom passive, the pace is brisk, yet within the pupils' capabilities, and where pupils learn to work independently and co-operatively with a sense of purpose. Clearly then, central to effective teaching is a focus on pupils' learning and pupils' engagement in learning, as well as the ability to be adaptable and to draw upon a range of skills and approaches to meet different situations and pupils' needs.

A number of personal qualities have also been associated with a good teacher such as enthusiasm, sense of humour, approachability, patience, impartiality, open mindedness, empathy, the ability to be a good communicator and organizer and to be caring towards pupils (Mawer, 1995; McNess et al., 2003; Larson, 2006). Pascual (2006) believes that:

> a good physical educator loves children, loves teaching. . .and is enthusiastic about the material
> s/he teaches . . . (p. 76)

Similarly, recent government policy documents in England (e.g. DfES/DCMS, 2004) have identified a number of characteristics of 'high quality' teachers. Examples include being committed, enthusiastic and positive role models, who listen to their pupils, raise their aspirations, and who improve their own subject expertise.

Effective teaching however, is not merely a matter of acquiring different skills and possessing certain personal qualities or characteristics, but also demands sufficient subject knowledge. Yet, this presents a particular challenge for physical education teachers who are required to teach across a wide variety of activities. Indeed, research has revealed that most trainee teachers are knowledgeable or feel confident or competent in teaching games, but lack knowledge in other areas such as dance, gymnastics, and outdoor and adventurous activities (Capel and Katene, 2000; Chedzoy, 2000; Gower and Capel, 2004; Sloan, 2007). Furthermore, subject knowledge for effective teaching comprises more than simply knowing the skills, tactics and rules of the different activities or one's content or subject matter. To achieve the skills required and which have just been highlighted demands teachers to have additional and broader knowledge such as general pedagogical knowledge (the broad principles and strategies of classroom management and organization applicable to teaching in general), pedagogical content knowledge (the combination of content and pedagogy that is the distinctive body of knowledge for teaching the subject and that makes it comprehensible to others), plus knowledge of the curriculum, the learners and the context.

Learning to Teach

Evidently there is much involved in becoming an effective physical education teacher. As you progress through your teacher training, first year of teaching, and beyond, you will progressively acquire the range of experiences to develop the skills required. Your development however, is unlikely to be smooth and linear but is likely to be characterized by many 'ups' and 'downs'. To help you to prepare and cope in this respect, it is worth considering how teachers develop and learn to teach and what aspects of learning to teach typically cause most anxiety.

It is commonly accepted that teachers learn to teach by experience but as they do so, they move through a number of developmental stages. Different models or stages of teacher development have been proposed over the years, two notable ones of which are outlined here (Fuller, 1969; Furlong and Maynard, 1995).

> ## Reflection
>
> Initially at this early stage of your teacher development:
>
> What concerns do you have?
> What is/are your most pressing concern/s?
> Compare your concerns with those of other trainees or newly qualified teachers or more experienced teachers
> Are there similarities and differences? If so, can you explain these?

Fuller (1969) presented a 'concerns based' model comprising three main stages of concern through which trainee teachers are reported to sequentially pass in their development as teachers. These include: self concern, task concern and impact concern. The first stage involves concerns about one's adequacy and survival as a teacher and includes concerns about, for example, class control, being liked and accepted by pupils and other staff, and fear of failure. When these initial self-concerns have been addressed the individual then becomes concerned about the task of teaching and concerns focus on the routine tasks that teachers are required to undertake. It is not until later that teachers become more concerned about meeting the needs of their pupils, the effect of their teaching on pupils' learning and development, and how they can enhance pupils' progress (i.e. impact concerns).

Since, and following on from the work of Fuller, a number of researchers have explored physical education teachers' concerns (e.g. McBride et al., 1986; Behets, 1990; Fung, 1993;

Hardy, 1996; Capel, 1998; Laker and Jones, 1998). In summary, trainee teachers' concerns relating to the following have commonly been reported:

- Subject knowledge
- Class management and organization
- Behaviour management
- Planning and preparation
- Pupils (e.g. pupil learning, motivation, enjoyment)
- School placement and expectations
- Acceptance/relationships with staff and pupils
- Persisting and/or coping with the demands of teacher training
- Being assessed/observed and receiving feedback

Of the above, behaviour management is often a particular pressing concern for trainees and indeed newly qualified teachers. This is probably heightened by frequent reports in the media about the discipline problems in schools, and by how adolescents are generally portrayed in the media and on television these days. Notable examples of the latter include Harry Enfield's moody teenage character 'Kevin', or Catherine Tate's modern day school girl 'Lauren' with her characteristic 'am I bovvered?' attitude. Be re-assured however, that such pictures do not represent the reality in the majority of schools, or for the majority of young people.

With respect to the process of learning to teach, Furlong and Maynard (1995) identified five broad stages in the development of trainee teachers:

Stage 1: early idealism

This stage occurs before trainees begin school experience and is characterized by clear but rather idealistic ideas, for example, about the sort of teachers they want to be, the kind of pupil relationships they wish to develop.

Stage 2: personal survival

At the start of school experience trainees' idealism fades when faced with the reality of the situation and they become concerned with their own personal survival. This involves them trying to 'fit in', with the major focus being on class control, class management and becoming established as a teacher.

Stage 3: dealing with difficulties

This stage occurs as trainees, having survived and adjusted to the realities of teaching, become sensitive to the different demands placed on them. They learn to make personal sense of what is happening in the classroom and, wanting to do well, often become focused on teaching methods and materials.

Stage 4: hitting a plateau

This occurs once trainees have gained basic competence and confidence in class and behaviour management and have identified what does and does not work. There is a tendency for them to 'stick to' what works, relax, and for their learning to hit a plateau. They often have trouble changing the focus from themselves to the needs of the pupils.

Stage 5: moving on

This occurs when trainees shift from focusing on themselves to their pupils and is when trainees are most successful, experiment with their teaching, and understand the need for change.

Clearly, these stages are not dissimilar to Fuller's concerns-based model whereby initially concern is with and about oneself (survival). Only when these initial self concerns have been addressed can the individual move on to address other aspects.

The implications

Possibly because of the complexity of the learning to teach process and the many factors involved, the results of research on the developmental stages of concern and learning to teach have been mixed, with some studies providing support or partial support for the stages and some not. Despite this, the models and their key principles serve as a useful guide and can be used to inform and support your teacher training and/or teacher development.

If you encounter different concerns and progress through different stages in your development as a teacher, then it follows that you will need different learning opportunities, experiences, targets, levels of support and challenge at different stages. In other words, and to maximize your learning, your training should similarly be developmental and your stages of concern and development at various points in time should be taken into account. For example, a trainee who is at the 'survival' stage is likely to require a great deal of support and guidance and experiences and targets which focus on developing fundamental teaching skills such as class management and organization and behaviour management, as well as on establishing routines, procedures and relationships. On the other hand, a trainee whose concerns have progressed beyond survival but who may have reached a 'plateau' is likely to benefit more from being challenged and given experiences, opportunities and targets with a pupil focus.

Assessment of Trainee and Newly Qualified Teachers

Earlier, being assessed was identified as a common concern for trainee teachers. Being aware of the expectations and requirements though, should help you to better prepare for, manage and progressively work towards and meet the demands of assessment without undue concern.

How specifically you will be assessed will be dependent on the context and/or nature of your teacher training or induction year, but it is likely to involve a range of methods and will involve an assessment of your practical teaching. In England, trainees' and newly qualified teachers' teaching is assessed against the Qualified Teacher Status (QTS) or the Core Standards respectively.

Professional Standards for Teachers in England

QTS is, at the time of writing, bestowed by the Department for Children, Schools and Families following an assessment which shows that a trainee has met all of the QTS Standards. Upon gaining QTS, the newly qualified teacher then begins an induction period by the end of which s/he must fully meet the Core Standards. The Standards are 'outcome' statements and are arranged in three inter-related sections covering:

- professional attributes;
- professional knowledge and understanding;
- professional skills.

Both sets of Standards form part of the Professional Standards Framework for teachers in England that was introduced in 2007. The Framework is progressive, defining the characteristics that teachers should demonstrate at each career stage, and provides Standards which progress from QTS through to Advanced Skills Teacher status. The intention is that the Standards and Framework be used to support teachers in identifying their areas of strength, development, and professional development needs to assist them in progressing to the next career stage.

Perhaps not surprisingly, national standards for teachers are not new or unique to England. For example, in the 1980s and 1990s educators in Australia, the United States and the United Kingdom began to consider what competencies a 'professional teacher' should demonstrate and to try to articulate these. However, there are critics of identifying specific competencies or standards for teachers who argue that they potentially fragment, technicize and decontextualize teachers' work, and to the contrary de-skill teachers and restrict their professional growth and development (Macdonald et al., 2006).

Assessment against the Standards

During your teacher training and induction period (and beyond), you will need to secure the necessary experiences to enable you to meet the relevant Standards and provide robust evidence that you have met them. Developing an understanding of the Standards, what is involved in meeting them, as well as a systematic method for monitoring and recording your g progress towards and achievement of them is therefore important. Early on, you will no doubt receive support with this from relevant tutors and staff. In addition, the TDA have produced guidance documents on the QTS Standards and the induction process for ITT providers, schools, trainees, and newly qualified teachers, as applicable (TDA, 2007a; 2007b), to support the understanding of and assessment evidence for the Standards.

Finally, and as acknowledged here, whilst working towards specific Standards may have limitations, try to focus on how they might be beneficial to you. For example, as a tool for monitoring your progress and securing the experiences and professional development you require, and for guiding review meetings and targets. After all, the QTS and Core Standards are only the beginning.

Learning More

Texts which provide further insight into physical education teaching and to some of the content addressed within this and subsequent chapters are available (e.g. Capel, 2005b; Green, 2008; Bailey and Kirk, 2009). In addition, there are some useful websites which provide relevant information and guidance to support your development as a physical education teacher (e.g. www.tda.gov.uk; www.afpe.org.uk).

References

Armour, K. (2006) Physical education teachers as career-long learners: a compelling research agenda, *Physical Education and Sport Pedagogy*, 11(3), pp. 203–207.

Bailey, R. (2005) *Teaching Physical Education: A Handbook for Primary and Secondary School Teachers*. London: Routledge (Taylor and Frances).

—(2009) Physical education and sport in schools: a review of the benefits and outcomes (pp. 29–38). In R. Bailey and D. Kirk (eds), *The Routledge Physical Education Reader*. London: Routledge (Taylor and Francis).

Bailey, R. and Kirk, D. (eds) (2009) *The Routledge Physical Education Reader*. London: Routledge (Taylor and Francis).

Behets, D. (1990) Concerns of pre-service physical education teachers, *Journal of Teaching in Physical Education*, 10, pp. 66–75.

Behets, D. and Vergauwen, L. (2006) Learning to teach in the field (pp. 407–424). In D. Kirk, D. Macdonald and M. O'Sullivan (eds), *The Handbook of Physical Education*. London: Sage.

Capel, S. (1998) A longitudinal study of the stages of development or concern of secondary PE students, *European Journal of Physical Education*, 3(2), pp. 185–199.

—(2005a) *Learning to Teach Physical Education in the Secondary School. A Companion to School Experience*. Second edition. London: RoutledgeFalmer.

—(2005b) Starting out as a PE teacher (pp. 6–18). In S. Capel (ed.), *Learning to Teach Phyisical Education in the Secondary School. A companion to School Experience*. Second Edition. London: RoutledgeFalmer.

Capel, S. and Katene, W. (2000) Secondary PGCE physical education students' perceptions of their subject knowledge, *European Physical Education Review*, 6(1), pp. 46–70.

Chedzoy, S. (2000) Students' perceived competence to teaching physical education to children aged 7 to 11 years in England, *Physical Education and Sport Pedagogy*, 5(1), pp. 104–127.

Department for Education and Skills and the Department for Culture, Media and Sport (2004) *High Quality PE and Sport for Young People. A Guide to Recognizing and Achieving High Quality PE and Sport in Schools and Clubs.* London: DfES.

Edmonds, S., Sharp, C. and Benefield, P. (2002) *Recruitment to and Retention on Initial Teacher Training: A Systematic Review.* Slough: NFER.

Evans, J. and Williams, T. (1989) Moving up and getting out: the classed and gendered opportunities of physical education teachers (pp. 235–251). In T. Templin and P. Schemp (eds), *Socialisation into Physical Education: Learning to Teach.* Indianapolis, IN: Benchmark Press.

Fuller, F.F. (1969) Concerns of teachers. A developmental conceptualization, *American Educational Research Journal*, 6, pp. 207–226.

Fung, L. (1993) Concerns among pre- and in-service physical educators, *Physical Education Review,* 16, pp. 27–30.

Furlong, J. and Maynard, T. (1995) *Mentoring Student Teachers: The Growth of Professional Knowledge.* London: Routledge.

Gower, C. and Capel, S. (2004) Newly qualified physical education teachers' experiences of developing subject knowledge prior to, during and after a postgraduate certificate in education course, *Physical Education and Sport Pedagogy*, 9(2), pp. 165–183.

Green, K. (2003) *Physical Education Teachers on Physical Education: A Sociological Study of Philosophies and Ideologies.* Chester: Chester Academic Press.

—(2008) *Understanding Physical Education.* London: Sage.

—(2009) Exploring the everyday 'philosophies' of physical education teachers from a sociological perspective (pp. 183–206). In R. Bailey and D. Kirk (eds), *The Routledge Physical Education Reader.* London: Routledge.

Hardy, C. (1996) Trainees' concerns, experiences and needs: Implications for mentoring in physical education (pp. 59–72). In M. Mawer (ed.), *Mentoring in Physical Education: Issues and Insights.* London: Falmer Press.

Kirk, D. (1992) *Defining Physical Education: The Social Construction of a School Subject in Postwar Britain.* London: Falmer Press.

Laker, A. and Jones, K. (1998) A longitudinal study of evolving student teacher concerns: baseline report, *Physical Education and Sport Pedagogy*, 3(2), pp. 200–211.

Larson, A. (2006) Student perception of caring teaching in physical education, *Sport, Education and Society*, 11(4), pp. 337–352.

Macdonald, D., Mitchell, J. and Mayer, D. (2006) Professional Standards for physical education teachers professional development: technologies for performance? *Physical Education and Sport Pedagogy*, 11(3), pp. 231–246.

Mawer, M. (1995) *The Effective Teaching of Physical Education.* Harlow: Longman.

McBride, R., Griffey, D.C. and Boggess, T.E. (1986) Concerns of in-service physical education teachers as compared to Fuller's concern model, *Journal of Teaching in Physical Education*, 5(3), pp. 149–156.

McNess, E., Broadfoot, P. and Osborn, M. (2003) Is the effective compromising the affective? *British Educational Research Journal*, 29, pp. 243–258.

Pascual, C. (2006) The initial training of physical education teachers in search of the lost meaning of professionalism, *Physical Education and Sport Pedagogy*, 11(1), pp. 69–82.

Siedentop, D. and Tannehill, D. (2000) *Developing Teaching Skills in Physical Education.* Fourth edition. Mountain View, CA: Mayfield Publishing Company.

Sloan, S. (2007) An investigation into the perceived level of personal subject knowledge and competence of a group of pre-service physical education teachers towards the teaching of secondary school gymnastics, *European Physical Education Review*, 13(1), pp. 57–80.

Training and Development Agency for Schools (2007a) *Professional Standards for Qualified Teacher Status and Requirements for Initial Teacher Training.* London: TDA.

—(2007b) *Supporting the Induction Process. TDA Guidance for Newly Qualified Teachers.* London: TDA.

Tsangaridou, N. (2006) Teachers' beliefs (pp. 486–501). In D. Kirk, D. Macdonald and M. O'Sullivan (eds), *The Handbook of Physical Education.* London: Sage.

Younger, M., Brindley, S., Pedder, D. and Haggar, H. (2004) Starting points: student teachers' reasons for becoming teachers and their preconceptions of what this will mean, *European Journal of Teacher Education,* 27(2), pp. 245–264.

The Practice of Physical Education and the Social Construction of Aims

David Kirk

Chapter Outline

The statement of aims and objectives was at one time the standard practice in education generally and in curriculum development more specifically. While the generality and content of aims differed, so that the aims of education in England might be more general than the aims of a specific subject such as physical education, or the aims of education in a particular school, nevertheless it was a matter of convention that the statement of aims came first, before detail of what the content of education might be, or the nature of specific learning experiences and how these might be assessed.

As a technology of curriculum development began to emerge first in the USA during the 1960s and later elsewhere, and as measurability of educational outcomes became a growing concern, objectives usually indicated a more detailed and substantive statement of educational intentions (Taba, 1962). The invention of behavioural objectives allied to approaches such as programmed learning (e.g., Magar, 1962) represented a high-point for some and a point of absurdity for others in the curriculum development process (Popham, 1970; Barrow, 1984). In the case of the former, the statement of educational intentions in the form of specific behaviours, that is, what learners will be able to do, held out a hope for the development of a scientific base for education. In the case of the latter, behavioural objectives were so detailed and concrete that their relationship to the broader aims of education was unhelpfully obscure and, so it was said, lost sight of the bigger picture.

It might be argued that curriculum development never really recovered from the shift towards behavioural objectives. Certainly, the idea that aims should be stated as a matter of first principle seems to have gone out of fashion for the planners and writers of school curricula nowadays, a trend that I will suggest may not actually be helpful. By way of example, in England and Wales, the National Curriculum as a whole has aims, but there are none stated for specific subjects as part of the *statutory* requirements (though aims do appear in the non-statutory advice to teachers – more of this shortly). Perhaps it could reasonably be argued that the technologization of curriculum development evidenced in the shift towards specific and measurable objectives created a culture over time in which the statement of aims was mistrusted and misunderstood. At the same time, the considerable variability of aims-talk, even within specific subjects such as physical education, inevitably contributed to this misunderstanding of what aims are and why we might find them useful.

It is to the nature of aims-talk that we turn first in this chapter, to examine the kinds of aims that have been stated for physical education and to see what they have in common and what makes them different. We then consider how aims are socially constructed in practice. A brief investigation of past and current practices reveals that the clear statement of aims, while making explicit assumptions and values, does not mean these will be implemented faithfully. What people say and do in the name of physical education in the present provides a context for understanding what it might be possible to aim for in the future. So, while we will argue that the current fashion for not stating aims is unhelpful since it risks leaving assumptions unexamined, the formerly common practice of stating aims as the first principle of curriculum development was also unhelpful. I propose instead that aims should be stated but only after we have carried out a careful study of current practice and how it is influenced by the residue of the past, a deceptively simple suggestion that has rarely been heeded by curriculum developers in physical education.

Aims-talk in Physical Education

Reflection

Before continuing with reading this chapter, reflect on and write down what you believe to be the aims of physical education. Return to these and consider them again once you have read the chapter. Would you change them, or would you leave them in their original form?

Although writing originally in the early 1950s, by the mid-1960s Randall (1967) was already able to note a considerable variety of aims-talk in physical education, ranging from the mainly physiological ('to be able to do the work of the day without undue fatigue' – quoting American McCloy), to the philosophical (physical education is education *of* the physical and *through* the physical), where the contribution physical education made to education more generally was included. This latter point was important for Randall himself. He adopted the advice of E.H. Le Maistre that there should be immediate objectives, general aims and an ultimate aim for physical education. Randall's immediate objectives were 'the development of skills'and 'enjoyment and satisfaction', general aims 'love of activity in the open air', 'love of physical exertion and the development of stamina', 'sense of values and desirable social attitudes', and 'good erect and well-developed physique', with the ultimate aim of 'optimum development of a balanced personality, mind and physique' (Randall, 1967, p. 45). Behind Randall's ultimate aim we can detect a holistic view of education captured in the Roman proverb *mens sana in corpore sano* ('a healthy mind in a healthy body') that informed the English Public School cult of athleticism (Mangan, 1981).

Reviewing more recent aims-talk, Laker (2000) noted a similar variability in the actual aims stated by different authors, but also some consistencies. For example, Willgoose (1984) in the USA focused on physical fitness, motor skills, social competency and intellectual competency as his four aims of physical education. Underwood (1983) writing around the same time in England stated that the five aims of physical education should be skill acquisition, education for leisure, health and fitness, socialization and enjoyment. Even though the language used is sometimes different, conveying a different emphasis according to each author's preferences, the development of the skills commonly understood to be prerequisites of participation in sports and games, physical fitness, and social attitudes or socialization seem to be mentioned regularly in aims-talk, while 'enjoyment' appears to be an enduring British focus, appearing in the statements of both Randall and Underwood.

More recently still, the following list of 'aims and purposes' of physical education at Key Stages 3 and 4 appeared on the Standards Site of the Department of Children, Schools and Families (2009) as non-statutory advice to teachers within the context of designing Schemes of Work based on the National Curriculum Physical Education (NCPE):

PE offers opportunities for pupils to:

- Become skilful and intelligent performers;
- Acquire and develop skills, performing with increasing physical competence and confidence, in a range of physical activities and contexts;
- Learn how to select and apply skills, tactics and compositional ideas to suit activities that need different approaches and ways of thinking;
- Develop their ideas in a creative way;
- Set targets for themselves and compete against others, individually and as team members;
- Understand what it takes to persevere, succeed and acknowledge others' success;
- Respond to a variety of challenges in a range of physical contexts and environments;
- Take the initiative, lead activity and focus on improving aspects of their own performance;
- Discover their own aptitudes and preferences for different activities;
- Develop positive attitudes to participation in physical activity.

This list of 'aims and purposes' of physical education is rather more specific than either of Underwood's or Willgoose's and is of course considerably longer. There is a level of detail here that readers familiar with the NCPE will find reasonably easy to map on to the statutory documentation. We can also see the reason why aims-talk might be treated with some mistrust and misunderstanding, by comparing the four lists of aims (Randall, Willgoose, Underwood and the DCSF), given the variability not only of the aims themselves but also of their relative generality.

Reflection

Reflect on the aims stated by the Department of Children, Schools and Families (2009). What values and beliefs do you think they express? In particular, what do you think the authors believe about physical activity, young people, and schools?

A final recent example of aims-talk for physical education at the level of an individual school shows that it is not just academic writers and government departments that engage in this practice. Arrow Vale Community High School (2009) states three 'school aims' and three 'community aims' for physical education:

> School Aim One
> . . . To improve the quality of teaching and learning in physical education and sport.
> School Aim Two
> . . . To insure that inclusion for all within physical education and Sport is achieved.
> School Aim Three
> . . . To develop the use of Information and Communication Technology within PE and Sport.
> Community Aim One
> . . . To provide a research and teacher centre for PE and Sport within the community.
> Community Aim Two
> . . . To provide a coaching and training programme for the pupils, students and the broader community.
> Community Aim Three
> . . . To develop vocational links within the community.

These aims are of a different kind to the other examples we have looked at, since they are less about the nature of physical education and more about the implementation and improvement of the subject, clearly and appropriately concerned with very local matters in school and community. In other words, while the other aims effectively seek to say something about what physical education *is* as a school subject, the Arrow Vale aims accept the nature of physical education as given (as indeed it is, in terms of the NCPE), and seek instead to state the school's intentions concerning specific aspects of the subject such as teaching and learning, inclusion and the use of technology.

This example reveals two important aspects of aims-talk. The first is that different kinds of statement can fall within the category of aims, which may be one of the reasons for the apparent retreat over the past two decades or more from stating aims as a first principle in discussions of education and the curriculum. While some curriculum development theorists have valiantly tried to set criteria for the use of the words 'aim', 'objective' and 'behavioural objective', they have not always been heeded by the writers of aims and objectives. The second is that in their most common form, and unlike the case of Arrow Vale, statements of aims are very much about offering definitions of a subject. This is a highly significant and often misunderstood point about aims-talk. We have looked at only a couple of examples of aims of physical education and there are many, many more. Each statement expresses particular preferences and priorities for physical education, making visible the particular values of the author. While some statements share words or notions in common, they also differ, sometimes to an alarming degree if we are at all concerned about reaching some measure of consensus on the nature of physical education as an educational activity.

Aims of the most common type found in educational literature tend then to state a preferred definition of a subject such as physical education. They are, in this context, statements of intention or purpose, in terms of saying not only what we value but what physical education seeks to achieve. Aims statements not only define the subject, in more or less explicit ways suggesting what the content will be and what students will learn, they also attempt to justify the subject, in terms of saying what physical education is for. Aims statements that are supported by careful, informed discussion such as is the case with Randall (1967) are helpful insofar as they provide a more or less clear statement of what we value, what we want to achieve, and why what we value and want to achieve are important.

But we would be quite wrong to suppose that by stating aims clearly and with justification that these statements might ever describe what actually happens in practice.

The Practice of Physical Education and the Social Construction of Aims

By stating their preferred aims of physical education, there are few authors who are naïve enough to imagine that these aims will be achieved easily or unproblematically. At the same time, most would hope, no doubt, that teachers might at least come close to realizing the aims and some would most certainly like to see teachers held accountable for doing so. This apparent gap between a statement of aims (or 'theory' as these might be known colloquially) and the reality of practice is well-enough known in the education field to be expected, even taken-for-granted. But this is not in fact the matter at hand.

If we want in the first place to understand the nature of physical education, of what physical education *is* and *is for*, examining a list of aims such as the DCSF's (2009) can only take us so far. Most aim-writers would, I suspect, accept this point, and would say that aims merely provide a starting point for curriculum development. However, the lessons that can be learned from curriculum history show that starting with aims as the first principle is premature. If we want to know what physical education might possibly achieve rather than merely what any particular individual or organization (even a government department) might prefer, we need to know what it is that teachers and students do and say in the name of physical education. Curriculum history suggests that physical education is socially constructed, so that what takes place in the name of physical education in any given place at a given time is the product of struggles over preferred values and priorities between what curriculum historian Ivor Goodson (1997) describes as coalitions of interested parties.

Reflection

Consider the aims listed by the Department of Children, Schools and Families (2009) in the previous section. What kinds of teaching and learning activities would occur in physical education in order to realize these aims? What kinds of things would teachers and pupils do in order to 'become skilful and intelligent performers' or to 'discover their own aptitudes and preferences for different activities'? Do current physical education programmes, in your experience, match these activities?

Past Practice

For example, during the period from the late 1800s to the early 1940s and prior to compulsory secondary education, physical training (as it was then known) for children attending government elementary schools in Australia and Britain consisted of what I have called 'drilling and exercising' (Kirk, 1992; 1998). Practices varied in different areas and indeed between schools in the same cities. But the distinctive features of this form of physical education were elements of military drilling such as marching and organizing in rank and file, mixed with elements of Dano-Swedish gymnastics. While the Department of Education's 1933 Syllabus of Physical Training in England sought to broaden physical education in government schools by including a whole chapter on 'The Organisation and Coaching of Games', a host of factors such as lack of playing fields and a lack of specialist teachers conspired to make such intentions difficult to implement, at least as a regular feature of the curriculum.

This important Syllabus, innovative in many ways, introduced a new aim for physical education that went beyond drilling and exercising. It was intended that *all* children rather than only those attending private schools should learn to play games and in so doing develop those aspects of 'character' central to the games ethic. However, the lack of more facilities and teachers was only one of the reasons that made achievement of this aim difficult (Mangan, 1981). There were also the prevailing expectations of teachers and education authorities, pupils, their parents and the general public, established over many years, that determined what aims were feasible to propose and possible to realize.

Teaching centred on drilling and exercising was intended to maintain discipline, to work on children's bodies in formal, precise and oftentimes tedious ways in order to regulate them, to maintain the standards of behaviour that schools required in order to function (Kirk, 1999). Children also had to become productive workers and parents, and drilling and exercising sought to instil obedience on the one hand, but a certain level of physical capability on the other. To be sure, these aims and expectations were by the 1940s somewhat out of date, having been established between the 1860s and the early 1900s, when compulsory schooling was for a generation of pupils a novel proposition. Nevertheless, they continued to exert an influence residually for many years after their replacement as official aims for physical education.

The matter of introducing games into physical education for government school pupils was further complicated not only by the fact that many stakeholders believed gymnastics to be the core of the subject, but also that there were different versions of gymnastics vying for a place in the curriculum. Swedish gymnastics, known also as Lingian gymnastics, was preferred by the British government in the late 1800s over several other versions, including the German *Turnen*, which was later to form the basis of competitive Olympic gymnastics. Interest in *Turnen* lay dormant in Britain during the first half of the twentieth century, although it was popular in physical training for boys between the middle to the end of the nineteenth century due to adaptations made by Archibald Maclaren and disseminated through the British Army Gymnastic staff (Major, 1966). Interest was re-kindled among the wider profession of physical educators following the 1948 London Olympics. At the same time, Rudolf Laban's work underpinned the innovation of educational gymnastics, championed by female physical educators in the 1940s through to the 1960s as an alternative to both Swedish and German gymnastics and enshrined as official government policy for primary school physical education in the early 1950s through the publication of *Moving and Growing* and *Planning the Programme* (Kirk, 1992).

Children in government schools did eventually experience the major games of netball, cricket, hockey, football and rugby as part of their regular physical education lessons, but not until the mid-to-late 1950s. Ironically, but not surprisingly given the historical roots of physical education in gymnastics, very few children actually got to learn to play games as such, and spent much of their lesson time learning the techniques required to play games. This skill-based approach to physical education teaching was justified by the claim that skills were prerequisites to playing a game (a matter that continues to be contested today). It was said that there was sufficient time in lessons only for skills and that pupils who were competent and interested could develop their abilities in extracurricular sport. As Whitehead and Hendry (1976) revealed, any teacher could supervise games play so long as they knew a little about the game, whereas only a qualified physical education teacher could teach skills.

As we now know with the benefit of hindsight and the Teaching Games for Understanding (TGfU) movement (Oslin and Mitchell, 2006), this focus on the techniques of games rather than game play was inappropriate and wrong if the aim of providing games in government schools was to produce good players. But once again what was possible had to be tempered by people's expectations and established practices. Teaching skills in parallel lines (rank and file), passing balls back and forward, or in drills that require order and organization, perpetuates the perception that physical education is concerned with the social surveillance and regulation of children's bodies. This in the 1950s and 1960s was an entirely reasonable position for teachers to take, given that eminent writers such as A.D. Munrow (1963) in *Pure and Applied Gymnastics* had sought to argue that drills and practices for teaching the skills of games were actually applied gymnastics.

The practice of physical education, what teachers and pupils do in the name of physical education, is a means of identifying the aims and purposes of the subject. So what does this tell us about current aims and what we might aim to do in the future?

Current Practice

Green et al. (2005) suggest that the establishment of the NCPE in England and Wales in 1988 and the various revisions since then have done little to change the dominant position of skill learning for games and sports. Moreover, even though additional activities have been added to the NCPE over the years since the late 1980s for girls and boys and that some girls express a preference for playing traditionally male games such as football (Flintoff and Scraton, 2001), physical education in practice in England and Wales remains the most sex-differentiated subject in the secondary school. This means that boys continue in the main to play football, rugby, cricket and basketball while girls are most likely to participate in hockey, netball, dance and aerobics (Green et al., 2005). While noting this continuity from practices established in the 1950s and 1960s, Green et al. (2005) are also careful to point out that the actual practice of physical education varies between schools, so that in some cases girls may in fact spend more time than boys in active participation in sports and games, and that in other schools boys may actually dance and play netball.

Adding the pupil's perspective to this analysis, Smith and Parr (2007) provide further evidence to reinforce Green et al.'s arguments about continuity. Pupils noted differences in their experience of physical education in Key Stage 3 where there was a particular emphasis on learning the prerequisite skills of games (which was relatively unpopular since the pupils found this repetitious) in comparison to Key Stage 4 where they actually played games and where they had some level of choice over activities (which was relatively popular). More generally, Smith and Parr found that pupils' experiences of physical education led them to say in interviews and focus groups that it provided them with a break from academic study (for those not taking GCSE physical education) and the opportunity for enjoyment and socializing with friends. While the pupils could recite the importance of physical education as a means of maintaining their health, Smith and Parr claimed the pupils' understanding of this connection was relatively superficial. The pupils had also absorbed the notion that physical education was a means of preparing for active leisure in adulthood, though there was a considerable diversity of views with respect to whether they personally saw this as a credible feature of physical education.

Taken together with the many other studies they cite, Green et al.'s and Smith and Parr's papers provide powerful insights into the social construction of contemporary physical education. Given a past dominated by gender-differentiation, by skill learning and by the surveillance and regulation of pupils' bodies dating from the drilling and exercising form of the subject, there has been a remarkable level of continuity in the practice of the subject despite the proliferation of aims over many years. At the same time, there has as Green et al. note, been change, in terms for example of the academicization of the subject through GCSE and A Levels and, we might add, through degree-level qualifications for teachers, an expansion of the curriculum to include more activities, and some evidence of a shift in the gender-orientation of the subject (though not uniformly across England and Wales).

Reflection

Write some aims that you think would fit actual physical education programmes as these are reported by Green and his colleagues, and Smith and Parr. Consider the curriculum, and what teachers and pupils say, and then write aims that accurately reflect these research findings rather than the official aims embodied in the NCPE or those listed by the Department of Children, Schools and Families (2009). Or do the official aims match these researchers' reports on current forms of physical education?

Conclusion: Aiming for the Future?

If what people say and do in the name of physical education effectively define the subject, it would appear to be important to know how physical education is socially constructed as a starting point for curriculum planning, rather than starting with the statement of aims as a first principle. While stating aims and supporting this statement with a rationale can be a valuable process of making explicit values and assumptions, I want to suggest that these aims need to be informed by an understanding of past and current practices and what might be possible in light of these practices. In the case of the evidence examined briefly of what teachers and pupils in some schools in England and Wales say and do in the name of physical education, we might conclude that the residual influence of the past remains strong in the present. At the same time, it might also be said that this influence continues at a reflexive or subconscious level, at the level of 'tradition' and assumption.

In more practical terms, all of this is to suggest that it may be helpful to state aims as part of the curriculum development process, as we seek to plan for the future. The apparent trend away from stating aims may leave the assumptions and values that inform curriculum construction implicit and unexamined. As I have argued, stating aims with a clear rationale not only forces us to think through what it is we are trying to achieve and whether these aspirations are feasible and reasonable, this also brings to the surface assumptions and values we hold. More than this, the statement of aims effectively defines the subject by stating explicitly what physical education *is* and *is for*.

However, and this is my key point, aims should not be the starting point of the curriculum development exercise. What comes first should be instead an investigation of the state of play, of current practices and the residual influence of the past. Such an investigation might in another context be called 'research', or at least, 'scholarship'. It is this practice, of carrying out a scholarly investigation ahead of stating aims and developing new curricula for the future, that curriculum developers invariably ignore. Scrutiny of any of the government's and its agents' physical education curriculum initiatives in the past two decades will show clearly that they have aimed for the future without understanding the present and past. This prevalent neglect of research as an essential aspect of the curriculum development process has resulted in initiatives that have made little difference to practice and produced the continuity of out-dated practices highlighted by Green et al. Even when aims are stated clearly and with a sound rationale, they must be informed by an understanding of where we are now and how we got here before we can have any reasonable hope of producing a form of physical education that will be well-suited to young people's needs in the future.

Learning More

Green (2008) provides a comprehensive introduction to a range of issues that shape the aims of physical education. Further information on the history of physical education since the Second World War can be found in Kirk (1992), while Penney and Chandler (2000) assist us to consider the future of the subject. There are a number of sources of information on contemporary forms of physical education from the perspectives of students (Green et al., 2005; Smith and Parr, 2007) and teachers (Williams and Bedward, 2001).

References

Arrow Vale Community High School (2009) http://www.arrowvale.worcs.sch.uk/sportscollege/peaims.htm (accessed: 21 January 2009).

Barrow, R. (1984) *Giving Teaching Back to Teachers: A Critical Introduction to Curriculum Theory*. Brighton: Wheatsheaf.

Department of Children, Schools and Families (2009) http://www.standards.dfes.gov.uk/schemes2/Secondary_PE/teachers_guide/section_one/aims/ (accessed: 21 January 2009).

Flintoff, A. and Scraton, S. (2001) Stepping into active leisure? Young women's perceptions of active lifestyles and their experiences of school physical education, *Sport, Education and Society*, 6, pp. 5–22.

Goodson, I.F. (1997) *The Changing Curriculum: Studies in Social Construction*. New York: Peter Lang.

Green, K. (2008) *Understanding Physical Education*. London: Sage.

Green, K., Smith, A. and Roberts, K. (2005) Young people and lifelong participation in sport and physical activity: a sociological perspective on contemporary physical education programmes in England and Wales, *Leisure Studies*, 24, pp. 27–43.

Kirk, D. (1992) *Defining Physical Education: The Social Construction of a School Subject in Postwar Britain*. London: Falmer.

—(1998) *Schooling Bodies: School Practice and Public Discourse 1880–1950*. London: Leicester University Press.

—(1999) Embodying the school/schooling bodies: physical education as disciplinary technology (pp. 181–196). In C. Symes and D. Meadmore (eds), *The Extra-Ordinary School: Parergonality and Pedagogy*. New York: Peter Lang.

Laker, A. (2000) *Beyond the Boundaries of Physical Education: Educating Young People for Citizenship and Social Responsibility*. London: Routledge.

Magar, R.F. (1962) *Preparing Instructional Objectives*. Palo Alto, CA: Featon.

Major, E. (1966) The development of physical education in England during the present century with special reference to gymnastics, *Carnegie Old Students Association Conference Papers*, 1, pp. 1–9.

Mangan, J.A. (1981) *Athleticism in Victorian and Edwardian Public Schools*. Cambridge: Cambridge University Press.

Munrow, A.D. (1963) *Pure and Applied Gymnastics*. London: Bell.

Oslin, J. and Mitchell, S. Game-centred approaches to teaching physical education (pp. 627–651). In D. Kirk, D. Macdonald and M. O'Sullivan (eds), *Handbook of Physical Education*. London: Sage.

Penney, D. and Chandler, T. (2000) Physical education: what future(s)?, *Sport, Education and Society*, 5, pp. 71–87.

Popham, W.J. (1970) Probing the Validity of Arguments Against Behavioral Goals (pp. 115–124). In R.J. Kibler, L.L. Barker, and D.T. Miles (eds) *Behavioral Objectives and Instruction*. Boston, MA: Allyn and Bacon.

Randall, M. (1967) *Modern Ideas on Physical Education*. London: Bell.

Smith, A. and Parr, M. (2007) Young people's views on the nature and purposes of physical education: a sociological analysis, *Sport, Education and Society*, 12, pp. 37–58.

Taba, H. (1962) *Curriculum Development: Theory and Practice*. New York: Harcourt, Brace and World Inc.

Underwood, G.L. (1983) *The Physical Education Curriculum in the Secondary School: Planning and Implementation*. Lewes: Falmer.

Whitehead, N. and Hendry, L.B. (1976) *Teaching Physical Education in England*. London: Lepus.

Willgoose, C.E. (1984) *Curriculum in Physical Education*. Englewood Cliffs, NJ: Prentice-Hall.

Williams, A. and Bedward, J. (2001) Gender, culture and the generation gap: Student and teacher perceptions of aspects of National Curriculum Physical Education, *Sport, Education and Society*, 6, pp. 53–66.

3 Health-related Physical Education

Jo Harris

This chapter will review developments in health-related physical education within the school curriculum and draw upon research findings to discuss issues associated with the area. Health-related physical education, which may also be known as 'health-related fitness' (HRF) or 'health-related exercise' (HRE), is defined as:

> the teaching of knowledge, understanding, physical competence and behavioural skills, and the creation of positive attitudes and confidence associated with current and lifelong participation in physical activity. (Harris, 2000, p. 2)

The chapter begins with a succinct overview of the relationship between physical education and health, followed by consideration of physical education's role in public health, and how teacher expertise in this area is acquired and developed. The conclusion provides a summary of contemporary issues associated with health-related physical education.

Overview of the Relationship between Physical Education and Health

Concerns about Children's Health and Physical condition first led to the introduction of physical education, albeit in the form of prescribed exercises, into the education system in England. The benefits of physical education were later broadened to include improved mental capacity and social skills, and there was a shift in emphasis toward freer forms of developmental movement (Kirk, 1992). It was not until the 1980s that there was a return to health as a key objective of physical education expressed in the form of 'health-related fitness' and 'health-related exercise'. These approaches attempted to broaden the traditional, competitive team-sport orientated programme to include education about lifetime physical activity and provide fitness-related activities such as aerobics and circuit-training; this development was associated with a more holistic notion of health incorporating psychological constructs such as motivation and self-esteem (Biddle, 1987).

During the 1990s, the evidence supporting the benefits of regular physical activity was strengthened (USDHHS, 1996) which led to physical education's role in promoting lifelong physical activity becoming more widely accepted. Shephard and Trudeau (2000) consider the key goal of physical education to be the promotion of active, healthy lifestyles and Green (2002, p. 95) makes reference to physical education's 'taken for granted role in health promotion'. There is certainly a strong belief that physical education can affect leisure-time physical activity through positive activity experiences and exercise education (Vilhjalmsson and Thorlindsson, 1998). Given these views, it is not surprising that the promotion of physically active lifestyles has become an established goal of physical education (National Association of Sport and Physical Education (NASPE), 2004a; Qualifications and Curriculum Authority (QCA), 2007).

The development of national physical activity recommendations for children has been a significant outcome of the increased evidence of the positive benefits of physical activity (Biddle et al., 1998; Corbin and Pangrazi, 1998; NASPE, 2004b). However, their impact on physical education in England appears limited with little evidence of them being formally incorporated into programmes of study (Cale and Harris, 2005). Furthermore, many physical educators view their subject as predominantly skill-centred and games-focused (Green, 2000) and consequently physical education tends to focus on a limited range of physical activities, particularly competitive team games (Fairclough et al., 2002). The limited provision of lifetime activities within physical education may alienate some young people from the subject and possibly from physical activity participation outside of school and later in life (Stratton et al., 2008). Establishing a solid foundation for further and future engagement in physical activity requires educational and psychological approaches which focus on young people acquiring the appropriate understanding and behavioural skills to ensure physical activity becomes a routine part of their daily life (Fairclough and Stratton, 2005). These approaches are more likely to have a greater long-term impact than those focusing solely on the volume of physical activity accumulated in physical education classes or specific fitness outcomes. Whilst a fitness-oriented approach might seem a productive one for physical education, traditional fitness programmes have been shown to have serious limitations (Harris and Cale, 2006).

The first NCPE in England (1992) incorporated 'health' but only as a theme to be implicitly embedded across a range of activity areas (e.g. athletics, games). This approach was criticized for marginalizing the area, and Harris's (1995, 1997) research revealed that physical education's role in promoting health was neither universally accepted nor well understood. Later revisions of the NCPE have arguably strengthened support for a health-related focus within the subject

(Fox and Harris, 2003; Cale and Harris, 2005; QCA, 2007). However, whilst this seems promising, the development of a health orientation within physical education has previously been over shadowed by the powerful influence of competitive sport within the subject (Hargreaves, 2000). The Physical Education, School Sport and Club Links (PESSCL) Strategy in England (Department for Education and Skills (DfES) and Department for Culture, Media and Sport (DCMS), 2003) provides further evidence of the strengthening of the model of sport as physical activity (Fox et al., 2004).

This influence is exemplified by Leggett's (2008) study of health-related exercise (HRE) policy and practice in secondary schools in England and Wales which detected minimal change in the expression of health in physical education from 1993 to 2001, and revealed that many physical education teachers articulated a 'fitness for life' philosophy but their delivery of HRE was usually expressed in terms of a 'fitness for performance' discourse, dominated by testing and training. This is consistent with Harris's (1995, 1997) earlier finding that many health-related programmes were oriented more towards 'fitness for sports performance' than 'fitness for healthy lifestyles'. Similarly, Green and Thurston (2002) found that an ideology of sport had penetrated deeply into the core assumptions of both physical education teachers and government in relation to the promotion of health through physical education. Leggett (2008) proposed that the 1999 versions of the NCPE in terms of HRE were simply not radical enough to necessitate any change in school level practice and concluded that, by itself, the NCPE is not the most effective avenue for changing HRE practice in schools due to the ways in which official discourse is interpreted and recontextualized within the pedagogical field. Ward and colleagues (2008) also reported concerns about the expression of health within physical education given that most physical education teachers claimed to value health-related learning, yet some had no written scheme of work outlining the nature and progression of this learning, and most relied on sport and fitness-related contexts to deliver it (Ward et al., 2008).

A number of tensions clearly exist in the relationship between physical education and health. Whilst it is considered that 'health' has been marginalized within physical education and that somewhat disparate agendas exist for physical education and public health (Harris, 1997, 2003), there is also a concern that 'physical education' as a distinctive area of learning could be threatened within the bigger umbrella of 'health education' or 'physical health and well-being', as expressed in the afPE's (2008) response to an independent review of the primary curriculum in England. Thus, there is somewhat of a dilemma in terms of how closely physical education wants (or needs) to be associated with health.

Physical Education's Role in Public Health

Physical education's role in public health is based on the premise that it provides opportunities to be active, educates about and through physical activity ('learning to move' and 'moving to learn') and sets the foundation for lifelong physical activity. Evidence of the health benefits of physical activity for children, however, is weaker than assumed although the rationale for promoting physical activity with children is considered to be strong (National Institute for Health and Clinical Excellence (NICE), 2007a). There are only small but significant physical-health benefits (relating to obesity, type II diabetes and skeletal health) and moderate psychological-health benefits (particularly relating to self-esteem and depression) of physical activity for children (NICE, 2007a). Further, the tracking of physical activity from childhood/adolescence into adulthood is limited (NICE, 2007a), and interventions which have increased physical activity during physical education lessons have not always had a positive impact on out-of-school activity (Salmon et al., 2007; Stratton et al., 2008).

Despite this, there has been increasing government interest in physical activity's role in public health and schools have been identified as playing a key part in this (Fox et al., 2004; McKenzie, 2007). Physical education and school sport is considered particularly important in terms of educating and providing opportunities for young people to become independently active for life (DfES and DCMS, 2003), and thereby helping to combat increases in sedentary behaviour and obesity. Indeed, school-based intervention studies have been shown to positively influence young people's health, activity and fitness levels, as well as their knowledge, understanding and attitudes towards physical activity (Harris and Cale, 1997; Stone et al., 1998), and the most effective children's physical activity interventions in the school setting have included some focus on physical education, in addition to activity breaks and family strategies (Salmon et al., 2007).

It is important, however, to be realistic about what physical education can achieve given that it has a range of objectives, only one of which is the promotion of physical activity (NASPE, 2004a; QCA, 2007). In addition, curricular physical education represents less than 1 per cent of a young person's waking time (Fox et al., 2004) and at least half of physical education lesson time can justifiably involve light or physically passive activity (Fairclough and Stratton, 2005, 2006; Stratton et al., 2008). One also has to be realistic about the numerous factors within and beyond the school setting which influence children's physical activity and the complexities involved in changing health behaviours (NICE, 2007b). It is known, for example, that knowledge and understanding of the importance of an active lifestyle is not sufficient to inspire young people to be physically active (Smith and Biddle, 2008). So clearly physical education cannot by itself address physical activity needs (Fox et al., 2004) or be held solely responsible for improving the health, activity and fitness status of young people. Furthermore, many countries around the world have witnessed a decrease in physical education time (Hardman and Marshall, 2005) although, exceptionally, physical education time in England has increased (OfSTED, 2005). However, more physical education time does not necessarily equate to increased attention to health and fitness. Indeed, the physical education profession in England has been criticized for paying insufficient attention to health and fitness (OfSTED, 2004) leading to weaknesses in many pupils' knowledge and understanding of this area (OfSTED, 2005, p. 1). This may contribute towards known misconceptions about health, activity and fitness amongst young people (Harris, 1993, 1994; Kulinna and Zhu, 2001; Placek et al., 2001; Stewart and Mitchell, 2003).

Physical education clearly needs to do what it can in the time available to it to contribute to the promotion and adoption of healthy, active lifestyles. In this respect, its key role should be to stimulate interest, enjoyment, knowledge and expertise in physical activity and sport for health and well-being (Fox et al., 2004). Suggestions for achieving this include: modifying instructional and organizational strategies to maximize student's 'active' learning; embracing more inclusive, student-centred curricula that place greater emphasis on lifetime physical activity; and leading whole-school approaches that make physical activity promotion a collective responsibility for teachers, students, parents, coaches and youth leaders (Stratton et al., 2008). To be truly effective, 'school physical activity promotion needs to expand from a restrictive, one-dimensional focus on traditional curricular physical education and sport to a model in which the culture and policy of the school is child-centred and health- and activity-driven' (Fox et al., 2004, p. 344) – as exemplified in the 'active school' model (Cale, 2000; Fox and Harris, 2003). Adopting an 'active school' approach though is challenging given the context of multiple demands on teachers, competing educational objectives, and the need for new skills among teachers (Fox et al., 2004). These whole-school approaches are also likely to be more effective if they are informed by improved understanding of the place and significance of physical activity in young people's lives (Wright et al., 2009), and of the views of young people about the barriers and facilitators to participation in physical activity (NICE, 2007b).

Reflection

In England, an identified area for development for primary and secondary schools has been 'increasing the amount of attention given to improving health and fitness in development plans' (OfSTED, 2004, p. 6). Weaknesses have been detected in many secondary school pupils' 'knowledge and understanding of fitness and health' (OfSTED, 2005, p. 1).

What do you think has contributed to 'health and fitness' being a relative weakness in school physical education?

Consider what actions could be taken to strengthen the focus on health and fitness.

Reflection

Young people have been shown to have incomplete and often inaccurate conceptions about health, activity and fitness (Harris, 1993, 1994; Kulinna and Zhu, 2001; Placek et al., 2001; Stewart and Mitchell, 2003). Examples include:

- Fitness is about looking good and being thin
- A particular exercise can reduce fat in a specific area
- Sweating will burn off fat
- Exercise involves hard work and being worn out
- Jogging improves strength.

How do you think that these (mis)conceptions have arisen?

What can be done to ensure that young people have a good understanding of health, activity and fitness?

Developing Teacher Expertise in Health-related Physical Education

The positive influence of professional development in health-related physical education has been demonstrated by studies showing that physical education specialists or classroom teachers who had received continuing professional development (CPD) (or both) engaged their students in significantly more moderate to vigorous physical activity than non-specialists or teachers who had not accessed CPD, through employing more efficient instructional methods and activity-promoting tasks (McKenzie et al., 1997, 2001). Another study demonstrated the positive impact of a HRE resource on many physical education teachers' knowledge, attitudes and confidence, and on their planning, content, evaluation, organization and delivery of HRE (Cale et al., 2002). However, it was less successful in changing teachers' philosophies and teaching methods which confirmed that resources by themselves are limited in their ability to bring about 'real' change – rather, they permit new ideas to be taken on board at a superficial level, or they are integrated within already well established philosophies and paradigms (Sparkes, 1994). A further positive example of HRE CPD is provided by Kulinna and colleagues (2008) who explored the impact of a year-long professional development intervention involving inexperienced teachers being paired with experienced teachers to help them learn how to teach a health-related physical education curriculum. The findings were supportive of the beneficial impact of this type of mentoring intervention on physical education teachers' psychosocial perceptions such as increases in attitude, perceived behavioural control, teaching behaviour and intention to teach fitness activity and activity-related knowledge.

For many physical education teachers, however, the reality is that 'health and life-long physical activity' do not feature in their professional development profiles (Ward et al., 2008). A national survey of secondary school teachers in England revealed that, for half of them, HRE had not been formally addressed within their initial training and over two-thirds had not participated in any HRE CPD in the previous three years (Ward et al., 2008). This limited engagement with health-related CPD along with the continued privileging of sport and fitness-related contexts was considered to result in less than effective delivery of health-related physical education (Ward et al., 2008). Furthermore, the professional development programme within the PESSCL Strategy in England (DfES and DCMS, 2003) revealed that 'health-related modules' were not selected by a high percentage of teachers – most primary teachers targeted modules associated with specific activity areas (e.g. gymnastics, games), and secondary teachers, whose take up of the modules was disappointingly low overall, did similar (Armour and Harris, 2008). This suggests that physical education teachers tend not to recognize their needs in relation to health-related learning – which may be due to their sports science background – it seems they believe they already know enough about this area and consequently choose not to prioritize it over other aspects of their work.

Yet, there is compelling evidence that physical education teachers do need CPD in health-related learning (Cardon and De Bourdeaudhuij, 2002; Cale, 2000) to face the challenge of 'acquiring the skills to promote "active living" particularly among those children who are disenchanted with traditional sport' (Fox et al., 2004, p. 351). Leggett (2008) also recommended health-related CPD to help teachers more closely match their practice with their philosophical perspective. Physical education teachers' need for health-related CPD is further demonstrated by the findings of a study which involved teachers taking a cognitive HRF test (designed for 13–15-year-olds) and a self-efficacy questionnaire (Castelli and Williams, 2007). The teachers were found to be over-confident about their knowledge of HRF – the vast majority thought that they would pass the test yet only just over a third did so. Castelli and Williams (2007, p. 13) considered it 'perplexing that many of the teachers were unable to design a physical activity programme appropriate for adolescent students' and stated that 'the revealed deficiencies in HRF knowledge among physical education teachers substantiate the findings of Miller and Housner (1998)', who found the HRF content knowledge of in-service and pre-service physical educators to be inadequate for effective teaching of health-related physical education. Thus, it would appear that physical education teachers' subject knowledge in HRF had not improved over this nine-year period of time. One possible explanation was ineffective professional development. However, Castelli and Williams (2008, p. 14) acknowledged, like others, that: 'Designing and providing teacher development . . . is difficult because few physical education teachers participate in professional activities . . . that would provide current information regarding HRF' (Zakrajsek and Woods, 1983). To this end, Castelli and Williams (2007) emphasized the need for pragmatic HRE resources alongside ongoing teacher development, particularly collaborative work between teachers and scholars to help bridge the research-to-teaching gap.

This leads one to wonder where physical education teachers are acquiring the professional subject knowledge they need to enable them to teach health-related physical education effectively? The findings suggest that, for the most part, they are not. Indeed, Armour and Yelling (2007) question whether physical education teachers will ever be in a position to demand the support they need in the interests of their pupils unless they accept greater responsibility for their role in promoting health through physical activity and/or are held more accountable for this (at the very least, within the school setting). Armour and Harris (2008) consider these to be important issues if health is to be a key focus of the work of physical educators, and they point to the tension between claims made for, and expectations placed upon, the subject in relation to public health – and its limited readiness/preparedness to deliver. For example, there is an expectation that schools can contribute to the reduction in childhood obesity by developing tailored programmes to increase participation in physical education and sport, and by creating a fresh set of programmes to ensure a clear legacy of increased physical activity leading up to and after the 2012 Games (DoH and Department for Children, Schools and Families (DCSF), 2008). However, Armour and Harris (2008) question who has the expertise to design and deliver these 'tailored', and 'fresh set' of, programmes? Or, indeed to create the 'world-class system of physical education and sport' designed to promote children's health and well-being to which the government in England has committed continued investment in CPD to equip teachers with the 'skills and expertise needed to inspire and engage all children and young people in physical education and sport' (HM Government, 2007, pp. 14–16). Armour and Harris (2008) propose that an important starting point for the physical education profession in this respect would be addressing uncertainties about: appropriate health knowledge for physical education; the 'proper' role for physical education in health; and the level of responsibility it should accept for health outcomes.

Conclusion

In summary, contemporary issues associated with health-related physical education are:

- High expectations of physical education to increase activity levels and reduce obesity amongst young people.
- A mismatch between many physical education teachers' 'fitness for health' philosophy and their 'fitness for performance' delivery of health-related physical education.
- Many young people's misconceptions about health, activity and fitness.
- Physical education teachers' over-confidence in their knowledge to teach, and limited engagement with professional development in, health-related physical education.

These are important issues which require attention as currently physical education is falling short of its potential contribution to public health and many physical education teachers are not well armed to meet the high 'health-related' expectations placed upon the subject.

Reflection

Consider how the issues summarized in the conclusion could be addressed by:

- National Associations for Physical Education (e.g. afPE; NASPE)
- Physical Education Teacher Educators
- Physical Education Leaders in Schools

Learning More

Further sources of information and guidance on health-related physical education are available for teachers (e.g. Cale and Harris, 2009) and for students and teacher-researchers (e.g. Cale and Harris, 2005). Some resources have been produced specifically to support whole school approaches to the promotion of healthy, active lifestyles (e.g. Department for

Education and Skills, 2006; Department of Health and Department for Education and Skills, 2007; www.healthyschools.gov.uk).

References

Armour, K. and Harris, J. (2008) Great expectations . . . and much ado about nothing? physical education and its role in public health in England. Paper presented at the American Educational Research Association Conference, New York.

Armour, K. and Yelling, M. (2007) Effective professional development for physical education teachers: the role of informal, collaborative learning, *Journal Of Teaching Physical Education*, 26(2), pp. 177–200.

Association for Physical Education (afPE) (2008) *Response to Review of Primary Curriculum*. www.afpe.org.uk (accessed: 15 December 2008).

Biddle, S. (ed.) (1987) *Foundations of Health-related Fitness in Physical Education*. London: Ling Publishing House.

Biddle, S.J.H., Sallis, J. and Cavill, N. (1998) *Young and Active? Young People and Health-Enhancing Physical Activity – Evidence and Implications*. London: Health Education Authority.

Cale, L. (2000) Physical activity promotion in secondary schools, *European Physical Education Review*, 6(1), pp. 71–90.

Cale, L., Harris, J. and Leggett, G. (2002) Making a difference? Lessons learned from a health-related exercise resource, *The Bulletin of Physical Education*, 38(3), pp. 145–160.

Cale, L. and Harris, J. (eds) (2005) *Exercise and Young People. Issues, Implications and Initiatives*. Basingstoke: Palgrave Macmillan.

Cale, L. and Harris, J. (2009) *Getting the Buggers Fit*. Second edition. London: Continuum.

Cardon, G. and De Bourdeaudhuij, I. (2002) Physical education and physical activity in elementary schools in Flanders, *European Journal of Physical Education*, 7(1), pp. 5–18.

Castelli, D. and Williams, L. (2007) Health-related fitness and physical education teachers' content knowledge, *Journal of Teaching in Physical Education*, 26, pp. 3–19.

Corbin, C.B. and Pangrazi, R.P. (1998) *Physical Activity for Children. A Statement of Guidelines*. Reston, VA: National Association for Sport and Physical Education.

Department for Education and Skills/Department for Culture, Media and Sport (2003) *Learning through PE And Sport. A Guide To The Physical Education, School Sport And Club Links Strategy*. London: HMSO.

Department for Education and Skills (2006) *Get Physical*. DVD, www.teachers.tv/getphysical

Department of Health/Department for Children, Families and Schools (2008) *Healthy Weight, Healthy Lives: A Cross-Government Strategy for England*. London: Department of Health.

Department Of Health and Department for Education and Skills (2007) *National Healthy Schools Programme. Physical Activity Toolkit. Booklets A and B*. London: Department of Health.

Fairclough, S.J. and Stratton, G. (2005) Physical education makes you fit and healthy. physical education's contribution to young people's physical activity levels, *Health Education Research*, 20, pp. 14–23.

—(2006) A review of physical activity levels during elementary school physical education, *Journal of Teaching in Physical Education*, 25, pp. 240–258.

Fairclough, S. J., Stratton, G. and Baldwin, G. (2002) The contribution of secondary school physical education to lifetime physical activity, *European Physical Education Review*, 8(1), pp. 69–84.

Fox, K., Cooper, A. and McKenna, J. (2004) The school and promotion of children's health-enhancing physical activity: perspectives from the United Kingdom, *Journal of Teaching in Physical Education*, 23, pp. 336–355.

Fox, K. and Harris, J. (2003) Promoting physical activity through schools (pp. 181–201). In J. McKenna and C. Riddoch (eds), *Perspectives on Health and Exercise*. Basingstoke: Palgrave Macmillan.

Green, K. (2002) Physical education and the 'Couch Potato Society' – Part One, *European Journal of Physical Education*, 7(2), pp. 95–107.

Green, K. and Thurston, M. (2002) Physical education and health promotion: a qualitative study of teachers' perceptions, *Health Education*, 102(3), pp. 113–123.

Hardman, K. and Marshall, J. (2005) Physical education in schools in European context: charter principles, promises and implementation realities (pp. 39–64). In K. Green and K. Hardman (eds), *Physical Education. Essential Issues*. London: Sage.

Harris, J. (1993) Young people's perceptions of health, fitness and exercise, *British Journal of Physical Education Research Supplement*, 13, pp. 2–5.

—(1994) Young people's perceptions of health, fitness and exercise: implications for the teaching of health-related exercise, *Physical Education Review*, 17(2), pp. 143–151.

—(1995) Physical education: a picture of health? *British Journal of Physical Education*, 26, pp. 25–32.

—(1997) Physical education: a picture of health? The implementation of health-related exercise in the national curriculum in secondary schools in England. Unpublished PhD thesis, Loughborough University.

—(2000) *Health-related Exercise in the National Curriculum. Key Stages 1 to 4.* Champaign, IL: Human Kinetics.

Harris, J., And Cale, L. (1997) How healthy is PE? A review of the effectiveness of health-related physical education programmes in schools, *Health Education Journal*, 56, pp. 84–104.

—(2006) A review of children's fitness testing, *European Physical Education Review*, 12(2), pp. 201–225.

HM Government (2007) *PSA Delivery Agreement 22: Deliver a Successful Olympic Games and Paralympic Games and Get More Children and Young People Taking Part in High Quality PE And Sport*. London: HM Treasury.

—(2008) *Healthy Weight, Healthy Lives: A Cross-Government Strategy for England*. London: HM Treasury.

Kirk, D. (1992) *Defining Physical Education. The Social Construction of a School Subject in Postwar Britain*. London: Falmer Press.

Kulinna, P.H. and Zhu, W. (2001) Fitness portfolio calibration for first through sixth-grade children, *Research Quarterly for Exercise and Sport*, 72, pp. 324–334.

Kulinna, P.H., McCaughtry, N., Martin, J.J., Cothran, D. and Faust, R. (2008) The influence of professional development on teachers' psychosocial perceptions of teaching a health-related physical education curriculum, *Journal of Teaching in Physical Education*, 27, pp. 292–307.

Leggett, G. (2008) A changing picture of health: health-related exercise policy and practice in physical education curricula in secondary schools in England and Wales. Unpublished Doctoral Thesis, Loughborough University.

Mckenzie, T. (2007) A public health perspective: for Pete's Sake! Paper presented at 'Historic Traditions and Future Directions in Research on Teaching and Teacher Education in Physical Education' Conference, Pittsburgh, USA.

McKenzie, T.L., Sallis, J.F., Kolod, B. and Faucett, F.N. (1997) Long-term effects of a physical education curriculum and staff development work: SPARK, *Research Quarterly in Exercise and Sport*, 68, pp. 280–291.

National Association for Sport and Physical Education (NASPE) (2004a) *Moving into the Future: National Standards For Physical Education*. Second edition. Boston: McGraw Hill.

—(2004b) *Physical Activity for Children: A Statement Of Guidelines*. Second edition. Reston, VA: Author.

National Institute for Health and Clinical Excellence (NICE) (2007a) *Physical Activity and Children. Review 1: Descriptive Epidemiology*. NICE Public Health Collaborating Centre: www.nice.org.uk.

—(2007b) *Physical Activity and Children. Review 3: The Views of Children on the Barriers and Facilitators to Participation in Physical Activity: A Review of Qualitative Studies*. NICE Public Health Collaborating Centre: www.nice.org.uk.

OfSTED (2004) *The School Sport Partnerships Programme: Evaluation of Phases 3 and 4 2003/04*. London: OfSTED.

—(2005) *Physical Education in Secondary Schools*. London: OfSTED.

Placek, J.H., Griffin, L.L., Dodds, P., Raymond, C., Tremino, F. and James, A. (2001) Middle school students' conceptions of fitness: the long road to a healthy lifestyle, *Journal of Teaching in Physical Education*, 20, pp. 314–323.

Qualifications and Curriculum Authority (2007) *Physical Education. Programme of Study. Key Stage 3. Key Stage 4.* www.qca.org.uk/curriculum.

Salmon, J., Booth, M.L., Phongsavan, P., Murphy, N. and Timperio, A. (2007) Promoting physical activity participation among children and adolescents, *Epidemiological Reviews*, 29, pp. 144–159.

Shephard, R.J. and Trudeau, F. (2000) The legacy of physical education: influences on adult lifestyle, *Pediatric Exercise Science*, 12, pp. 34–50.

Smith, A.L. and Biddle, S.J.H. (eds) (2008) *Youth Physical Activity and Sedentary Behaviour: Challenges and Solutions.* Champaign, IL: Human Kinetics.

Sparkes, A. (1994) Curriculum change: on gaining a sense of perspective. In N. Armstrong, and A. Sparkes (eds), *Issues in Physical Education.* London: Cassell.

Stewart, S. and Mitchell, M. (2003) Instructional variables and student knowledge and conceptions of fitness, *Journal of Teaching in Physical Education*, 22, pp. 533–551.

Stone, E.J., Mckenzie, T.L., Welk, G.J. and Booth, M.L. (1998) Effects of physical activity interventions in youth: review and synthesis, *American Journal of Preventative Medicine*, 15(4), pp. 298–315.

Stratton, G., Fairclough, S.J., and Ridgers, N. (2008) Physical activity levels during the school day. In A.L. Smith and S.J.H. Biddle (eds), *Youth Physical Activity and Sedentary Behaviour. Challenges and Solutions.* Champaign, IL: Human Kinetics.

United States Department of Health and Human Services (USDHHS) (1996) *Physical Activity and Health: A Report of the Surgeon General.* Atlanta, GA: Centers for Disease Control and Prevention.

Vilhjalmsson, R. and Thorlindsson, T. (1998) Factors related to physical activity: a study of adolescents, *Social Science and Medicine*, 47, pp. 665–675.

Ward, L., Cale, L. and Webb, L. (2008) Physical education teachers' knowledge and continuing professional development in health related exercise: a healthy profile? Paper presented at the British Educational Research Association Conference, Edinburgh, September 2008.

Wright, J., Macdonald, D. and Groom, L. (2009) Physical activity and young people. beyond participation. In R.P. Bailey and D. Kirk (eds), *The Routledge Physical Education Reader.* London: Routledge.

Zakrajsek, D. and Woods, J.L. (1983) A survey of professional practices: elementary and secondary physical educators, *Journal of Physical Education, Recreation and Dance*, 54(9), pp. 65–67.

Career-long Professional Learning for the Professional Physical Education Teacher

4

Kathleen Armour, Kyriaki Makopoulou,
Fiona Chambers and Rebecca Duncombe

Chapter Outline

'Teachers matter' (Cochrane Smith, 2005). More specifically, teachers' career-long professional learning matters. Why? Because over the course of a career, each individual teacher has the potential to make positive – or negative – impacts upon many thousands of pupils. It is a point worth emphasizing. For example, in a typical 35-year career, we estimate that each teacher will teach classes of approximately 30 pupils, 20–30 lessons per week, for approximately 40 weeks each year. Having performed the calculation, and even allowing for the wide range in individual career structures, the inescapable conclusion is that whereas 'every child matters' (i.e. in UK education policy), and no 'child [should be] left behind (in the US), such sentiments are meaningless if teachers' learning 'doesn't matter' with the result that they are 'left behind'. Cochrane Smith (2005, p. 6) points out that teachers' work 'makes a difference in children's lives, and we should pay more attention to policies and practices assuring that all children have good teachers'.

We argue in this chapter that one of the defining characteristics of a 'good' physical education teacher is a commitment to career-long professional learning. Moreover, as members of a profession, teachers are entitled to expect that their professional learning will be supported by effective policies and structures in schools and the wider physical education community of which they are a part. What this means for you upon entry to the teaching profession is that engaging in appropriate CPD cannot be regarded as optional. Instead, you need to view successful completion of initial teacher education as the *beginning* of a professional learning career. Indeed, we argue that engagement in effective CPD is the *only* way in which the physical education profession can ensure that teachers are acting in the best interests of the children and young people they exist to serve. Essentially, the nature and quality of teachers' learning matters for the quality of children's learning, so this chapter encourages you to consider physical education teachers not as teachers, but as *learners*. Each section that follows includes illustrative quotes from research undertaken in different countries with physical education teachers, and short tasks to guide you into becoming a teacher who learns.

On Being a Professional in Physical Education

> Louise was just coasting, she wasn't being challenged in any way in her job . . . I don't know how to deal with her because she is so bright and intelligent that really all her . . . talents are not being utilised properly . . . she had a PE inspection and that was the only reason that she had gone to in-service [CPD]. She hadn't attended in-service in many, many years.
>
> (An Irish head teacher commenting on a member of the
> PE department in his secondary school)

In most countries, teaching is considered to be a profession even though it is not always accorded the same status as some other professions (Shulman, 2000; Hargreaves et al., 2007). Etzioni (1969) famously referred to teaching as a 'semi-profession' because it lacks the professional autonomy and respect that are defining characteristics of established professions. In 1987, Pluckrose went even further arguing that teaching failed to qualify as a profession on four counts: lack of authority, confusion over the client (child, parent or society?), the absence of a unified professional body and the absence of agreed professional standards. In particular, Pluckrose identified exclusivity and specialized knowledge as key features of a true profession: 'A profession tends to have few members, each member possessing esoteric knowledge which sets him or her apart from their peers' (pp. 73–74). In 1997, Helsby et al. made the further distinction between *being* a professional and *behaving* as a professional. Clearly, any individuals or occupational groups could make the claim that they *behave professionally*; that is, in a manner regarded to be appropriate for members of a profession. *Being* a professional, however, is a rather more exacting claim that is dependent upon the completion of specified training and the award of qualifications that act as a filter into a professional occupation.

There is ample evidence that the terms 'profession' and 'professional' remain contested – as even a cursory search on Google will confirm. Moreover, as public imperatives and policies change over time, debates about what it means to be a profession change too. For example, since Pluckrose's arguments in 1987, there has been an increase in the deployment of professional 'standards' for teaching (Sato et al., 2008) which can be used to guide teacher learning through initial teacher training and into induction and beyond (Smith and Reading, 2001). There can be little doubt, however, that some occupational groups appear largely secure in their designation as a 'profession', suggesting there are few serious challenges to their status. Obvious examples of 'secure' professions include medicine and law. Other groups, such as teaching, continue to strive to make their case.

There have been numerous attempts to crystallize what it is that sets 'professions' apart from other occupational groups. Day (1999, p. 5) concluded that professions are distinguished by:

(i) a specialised knowledge base – technical culture;
(ii) a commitment to meeting client needs – service ethic;
(iii) a strong collective identity – professional commitment; and
(iv) collegial as against bureaucratic control over practice and professional standards – professional autonomy.

The Australian Council of Professions identified knowledge and ethics as key features of a profession, but also emphasized public recognition and moral responsibility:

A disciplined group of individuals who adhere to high ethical standards and uphold themselves to, and are accepted by, the public as possessing special knowledge and skills in a widely recognised, organised body of learning derived from education and training at a high level, and who are prepared to exercise this knowledge and these skills in the interest of others.

Inherent in this definition is the concept that the responsibility for the welfare, health and safety of the community shall take precedence over other considerations. (http://www.accc.gov.au/content/index.phtml/itemId/277772; accessed: 5 March 2009)

This latter definition appears to resonate strongly with the purposes of teaching, so it is interesting to note that the same website offers examples of professions, but does not select 'teacher' as one of them:

- health related – doctors, dentists, physiotherapists, podiatrists, pharmacists
- non-health related – architects, engineers, veterinarians, surveyors, lawyers

In referring to professions as 'disciplined', the Australian Council definition raises the issue of autonomy. Professional autonomy is a key characteristic of professions and it is defended fiercely, however, in order to retain autonomy, professions are expected to undertake rigorous internal critiques of their structure, purpose and effectiveness. As a result of such activities, and in restating their aims and commitments, professions are able to reassure internal and external communities about the steps they are taking to assure their professional 'health'. The case of the pharmacy profession is illustrative. In considering what it is to be a professional pharmacist, an article written for pharmacy students suggests that active engagement in continuing education is a pivotal requirement:

> If as a pharmacist you are going to perform your duties competently, then you will need to keep up to date with all aspects of professional practice . . . any new pharmacist, if they are to be a true professional, must embark on continuing professional education . . . *Continuing education involves more than passively attending a few courses, it involves the pharmacist taking some responsibility for his or her own learning.* Thus, as a pharmacist, you should approach continuing education in the broadest sense, using all available resources at your disposal. (Rees, 1999, pp. 24–26, our emphasis)

Brunetti (1998, p. 62) made a similar claim: 'a well developed, readily available continuing education programme is the hallmark of a true profession.' This leads us to important questions about teachers as learners and about CPD within the teaching profession.

Reflection

Does teaching qualify as a full profession? Consider the arguments for and against designating teaching as a profession by drawing comparisons with the claims made to professional status by other occupational groups. If you conclude that teaching is – or is not – a profession, what are the implications for physical education teachers?

On Professional Learning in Teaching

> *Most seminars are boring because we go there just because someone has told us to do so and we listen to things that we've heard some years ago. It is pointless. Each seminar is disconnected to previous seminars. I do not believe that we do anything different as a result.*
>
> (Secondary school physical education teacher in Greece evaluating his career-long CPD experiences)

> *The module, well it was partly helpful, because I knew many of these things already . . . I've been teaching for over 20 years and have been to other courses . . . so I only got one or two things out of it."*
>
> (Primary school teacher in England commenting on a CPD course in physical education)

Falk (2001, p. 137) claimed that 'professional learning is *the* job of teaching'. As an aspiration, this is clearly laudable. In practice, however, there is little evidence to suggest that teachers have routinely placed professional learning at the heart of their professional identities, nor that professional development structures have supported teachers to be active learners engaged in sustained and challenging professional learning (Wayne et al., 2008). James et al.

(2007, p. 217) in the conclusion to a major teaching and learning research project undertaken in England, argued that teachers need to move away from 'performing teaching' to 'supporting learning'. In addition, these authors argued that teachers who were most successful in supporting student learning were those who 'took responsibility for what happened in their classrooms. They were not inclined to blame external circumstances or pupil characteristics . . .' (p. 215). There are echoes in these findings of Dewey's (1958) call for dynamic professional teachers who are 'moved by their own intelligences and ideas' and Schon's (1971, p. 30) arguments for developing schools as 'learning systems, that is to say, systems capable of bringing about their own continuing transformation'. What all these points have in common is a view of schools and teachers as active in their professional growth and development; thus supporting Falk's aspirant view of professional learning as a core focus of teaching. So, what is known about the nature and structure of CPD for teachers?

Given the emphasis that is placed on CPD both in general definitions of 'professions' and in developing successful teachers, it is interesting to speculate on the rationale underpinning the provision of CPD that has prevailed in teaching. It is difficult to imagine a less effective CPD 'system' than the one that has operated in many countries to date; and physical education CPD is no exception. For example, traditionally, teachers' career-long learning has been characterized by sporadic one-day 'courses', on a series of topics disconnected from previous learning (often information-giving about the latest education policies), delivered out of the school context and with a group of teachers all of whom have different individual needs (differing career-stages, experience etc). These courses rarely have pupils present and are often designed without follow-up learning support (Craft, 2000), so although such courses can be useful and informative as one element of a broader CPD strategy, they are unlikely to be effective if they represent the *only* CPD strategy. Unsurprisingly, perhaps, there is now wide-spread agreement that this approach to teacher learning is likely to have limited impact on teachers' practices (Craft, 2000; Day and Sachs, 2004; Garet et al., 2001). Indeed, Borko (2004, p. 3) described much existing CPD for teachers as 'woefully inadequate', and as James et al. (2007, p. 63) argue: 'Advice on specific classroom practices may be useful in the short term but continuous and progressive professional development will have more lasting value.'

Elmore (2007) commented that continuous mastery of new knowledge should be a condition of practice for all teachers. He also argued that teachers have been too passive in the past and that they need to take a more active role in establishing and owning their professional practices. Yet research with physical teachers, as with other teachers, makes it apparent that they have long suspected CPD was inadequate for their needs. One of the most startling findings from research with ten case study physical education teachers, where we tracked all aspects of their professional learning over one academic year, was that the findings mirrored precisely the international research on effective/ineffective CPD (Armour and Yelling, 2007). In the absence of enabling CPD structures in schools underpinned by alternative visions of teacher learning, it is difficult to see what changes these teachers could have evoked; nonetheless, Elmore's point is worth considering. If it is the responsibility of a professional to seek out and engage actively in appropriate professional learning to meet clients' needs, as was argued in the pharmacy example cited earlier, and if physical education teachers were aware of the shortcomings of the CPD that was available to them, how has the ineffective CPD 'system' been perpetuated?

The answers to that question take us to the heart of this discussion. One answer might be that as a 'semi-profession' (Etzioni, 1969) teaching simply has not had the credibility or autonomy to develop CPD that would better meet its needs. Another answer might lie in Pluckrose's (1987) concerns that the 'client' in education is unclear and so the focus of CPD is similarly fuzzy (although to us it is entirely clear; it is the pupil). Another possibility, however, is that teachers tend to be viewed as just that – teachers – rather than learners. Thus, teachers are expected to go to work each day to **teach**, instead of to learn continuously about pupils' and their learning needs. It is a subtle distinction, but the outcome is that teaching and professional learning have, through traditional professional development structures, become fractured into two quite separate entities. As such, teaching and professional learning often occur in different locations and at different times instead of being treated as what they must surely be: two sides of the same coin.

It is this understanding of the unity of teaching and professional learning that underpins much of the contemporary research and literature on CPD generally and within physical education. In particular, research has striven to identify the characteristics of effective professional development. For example, Sparks (2002, pp. 1–4) defined effective CPD as that which:

- deepens teachers' content knowledge and pedagogical skills;
- includes opportunities for practice, reflection and research;
- is embedded in the workplace and takes place in the school day;
- is sustained over time; and
- is founded on a sense of collegiality and collaboration.

Similar findings emerged from an interesting study undertaken in the USA on case study schools that were failing in one or more aspects of provision. In these cases, enhanced professional development for teachers was placed at the centre of school improvement strategies. West Ed (2002, p. 12) entitled the report of their findings: 'Teachers who learn: Kids who achieve' and concluded that teacher learning is pivotal to school improvement and in order to make CPD effective, schools should:

- ensure that student-centred goals underpin all professional development;
- accept an expanded definition of professional development, embracing a wide range of formal and informal learning experiences;
- recognize, value and make space for 'ongoing, job-embedded informal learning';
- structure a collaborative learning environment;
- ensure there is time for professional learning and collaboration; and
- check (constantly) whether professional development is having an impact on pupils' learning.

Guskey (1994; 2002) argued that although more research evidence about CPD has become available, the profession still needs much better evidence about the effects of different forms of CPD on teaching, learning and student achievement. Importantly, Guskey reminds us that there is no single form of CPD that is appropriate for all teachers; what is required is an 'optimal mix' of activities that suits particular teachers at different stages in their individual development. In other words (and this shouldn't surprise us) teachers, like pupils, are not well served by CPD providers who attempt to 'deliver' one-size-fits-all learning. Thus, Guskey argued we need a paradigm shift in CPD. Instead of viewing teachers as passive learners, CPD should be viewed as an opportunity to help teachers to develop as independent thinkers and knowledge creators. Similarly, Day and Sachs (2004) identified two different models of CPD. The deficit model assumes that CPD providers must 'fill' teachers with knowledge that they lack; and this would appear to be the prevailing model to date. The aspirational model, however, acknowledges the need for teachers to engage in continuous learning within schools that value professional learning and that operate as school-wide learning communities. Clearly this view represents something of a departure from the traditional CPD 'courses' that many teachers have attended throughout their careers.

A further issue identified in the research on effective CPD by both Sparks (2002) and West Ed (2002) is learning context; essentially, context matters and embedding learning within 'real' teaching contexts is pivotal. It is apparent that teachers (like most learners) need considerable support to transfer information that is delivered in contexts very different to the ones in which they work (Penuel et al., 2007). For example, Cothran et al. (2006) conducted research into the ways in which physical education teachers in elementary schools in the USA responded to a mandated curriculum change that required them to focus on public health. The researchers found that although specific training for the change was made available, it was provided within a traditional 'one-off' course model with little follow-up support. After attendance at the course, teachers reported feeling overwhelmed; unable to learn all the information that was provided or to see its relevance to their own school contexts. Essentially, the teachers didn't feel that the knowledge they were given related well to the real world of teaching; so they rejected it. This leads to two important questions: what should teachers be learning in career-long CPD and how should that learning be structured?

Reflection

1. If it is accepted that the traditional 'course' led model of professional development is often ineffective in supporting teachers' learning, consider all the reasons why the model has endured. In particular, consider the advantages and disadvantages of the traditional model for teachers, schools and professional development providers.
2. Select a country in which you are interested and find out how professional development for teachers is organized and whether any research has been conducted to evaluate the strengths and weaknesses of the provision.

On Career-long Learning . . . but Learning What and How?

I mean some of the things that come through, I don't think are pitched at professional PE teachers now, as in somebody who has studied PE for four years and is a specialist PE teacher. I think a lot of professional development stuff that comes through is pitched at a lower level.

(Secondary school PE teacher in England commenting on the lack of challenge in PE CPD)

Day (1999) argued that CPD is about providing professionals with the skills and knowledge they need to be successful members of a profession. In some countries, national curricula and professional standards have been articulated and, at one level, it could be argued that these provide a basis for designing CPD. Certainly comprehensive professional standards can alert us to the complexity of teaching, thus confirming that teaching is about more than simply acquiring an adequate knowledge of the curriculum subject to be taught. Huberman (1983) defined the 'craft knowledge' of teaching as embracing a wide range of professional skills and Garet et al. (2001) summarize the range of professional development activities required as follows:

> Some activities are intended primarily to improve teachers' knowledge of subject-matter content; some are designed to improve general pedagogy or teaching practices, such as classroom management, lesson planning, or grouping methods; and some are intended to improve what Shulman (1987) has termed 'pedagogical content knowledge' – teaching practices in specific context domains, such as teaching multi-digit addition in elementary mathematics or forces and motion in physics. (p. 923)

Until recently there was very little research evidence available on what physical education teachers learn throughout their careers. However, research undertaken between 2001 and 2003 examined the career-long professional development profiles of a sample of physical education teachers in England (Armour and Yelling, 2004). In summary, the profiles illustrated that these teachers' CPD experiences were lacking coherence, relevance, challenge and progression. In terms of content, most of the physical education CPD undertaken consisted of sports update or coaching courses, undertaken sporadically over a career. It was also interesting to note that the CPD available to these physical education teachers failed to match up to the pupil learning outcomes that the teachers themselves identified as central to their programmes. In particular, there was little or no professional development available in health or personal/social development through sport or physical education. These findings were pursued further through in-depth case studies with ten physical education teachers, charting all the professional learning in which they were engaged over the course of one academic year (Armour and Yelling, 2007). From these teachers we learnt that although their

CPD histories were also dominated by traditional forms of CPD (i.e. one-off, off-site, sports coaching courses) they had strong beliefs about the value of learning collaboratively with and from professional colleagues; indeed they reported this to be the most valuable form of CPD. Ironically, these teachers were also aware that informal, collaborative learning wasn't viewed as 'real' CPD by their schools. On the other hand, if they attended an official CPD 'course' that required them to abandon their pupils for a day and that was, ultimately, ineffective, they were often able to count this as CPD by recording evidence of attendance as sufficient evidence of learning.

The Physical Eduction teachers in this research in England were not unusual. Research with teachers from around the world and in a range of curriculum subjects has reported similar findings. As Loughran and Gunstone (1997, p. 197) commented, teachers tend to view CPD with 'a healthy cynicism' as they 'wait to be convinced' that the time spent 'doing' professional development will be beneficial to themselves and their pupils. There can be little doubt, therefore, that this 'system' of CPD is unworthy of an occupation that claims to be a profession. It is a system which encourages CPD providers to offer identical courses to different teachers at different stages in their careers, who work in different schools and with different pupils who differ in their learning needs in all sorts of ways. Ironically, it is then expected that these same teachers will develop pupils into autonomous, lifelong learners by providing differentiated learning experiences and personalized learning in order to raise pupils' aspirations and meet their individual learning needs. All of this begs again the question that was raised earlier in this chapter – why has this ineffective CPD system survived for so long in a profession that is reputed to have learning at its core?

One reason for the endurance of the existing CPD system was explored earlier in this chapter: a lack of research on teachers' professional development, particularly in the field of physical education. Another reason has been offered by Mujis and Lindsey (2008): inadequate evaluation of CPD activities. Most evaluation – if it takes place at all – takes the form of surveys of teachers' opinions (opinionnaires) taken immediately after attendance at a CPD event. This approach tells us nothing about whether and how teachers use what they have learnt, and whether pupils' learning improves as a result . . . or, indeed, gets worse. This makes it impossible to determine whether public funds should be spent on CPD, or on particular types of CPD (Wayne et al., 2008). As Garet et al. (2001, p. 917) contend, there has been 'relatively little systematic research on the effects of professional development on improvement in teaching or on student outcomes'. Guskey (2000) raised similar concerns and argued that in order to be effective, evaluation needs to be undertaken at five distinct levels: participant support, participant learning, organizational support, participant behaviour and student learning outcomes. Moreover, it could be argued that only after undertaking evaluation at all five levels is it possible to make an estimate of value for money.

It is clear from the evidence presented so far in this chapter that there is a growing awareness of the importance of teachers' learning for the quality of pupils' learning; and there is an accumulation of research evidence identifying the characteristics of effective and ineffective CPD. In England, as elsewhere in the world, teachers' CPD has become increasingly prominent in education policy. In a major policy document in 2001, the UK government stated that CPD should represent 'good value' and that quality CPD should:

- meet individual, school or national development priorities;
- be based on good practice;
- help raise standards of pupil achievement;
- respect cultural diversity;
- be provided by skilled experts;
- be systematically planned;
- be based on relevant standards, current research and inspection evidence;
- make effective use of resources;
- be provided in sound accommodation; and
- include effective monitoring and evaluation systems (DfEE, 2001, p.1).

Identification of the need for monitoring and evaluation in this policy had an immediate and direct impact on physical education. As part of the English government's extensive PESSCL strategy (see http://www.sportengland.org/pesscl.htm for details), a new national physical education CPD programme was designed and launched in 2003, with (for the first time) accompanying funds allocated for evaluation research. The aims of the national CPD programme were broad:

- Improving the quality of teaching and learning in physical education and school sport in order to raise the attainment of all pupils
- Increasing the understanding of the use of high quality physical education and school sport in whole school improvement
- Enhancing the links between high quality physical education and school sport and the promotion of physical activity and health
- Encouraging innovative interpretation of the national curriculum for physical education to ensure it closely meets pupils' needs and ensures their maximum achievement.

The programme took the form of a series of 'modules'; some delivered as traditional 'courses', others as resources, that were designed nationally but delivered locally. Schools and teachers were required to undertake an audit of CPD needs before accessing modules and local CPD providers were appointed to ensure that provision matched teachers' and schools' needs. The modules were available free of charge to all teachers in all schools. In phase two of the programme, schools were encouraged to engage in innovative forms of CPD, for example, by creating local professional learning communities.

The findings from the evaluation research reinforced those from previous CPD and physical education CPD studies. For teachers, CPD was most likely to be regarded as effective when:

- two or more teachers from the same school attended a module together;
- the module was school-based, with 'my' pupils;
- the audit process led to appropriate module selection;
- trainers were able to adapt the modules to meet teachers' different needs;

- modules could be linked to school improvement plans;
- the learning was active and interactive;
- there was follow-up learning support; and
- collaborative professional learning was facilitated (Makopoulou and Armour, 2006; Armour and Makopoulou, 2008).

One of the key research findings, illustrated vividly in the case studies, was the value teachers placed on collaborative professional learning, and this echoes earlier physical education research (Armour and Duncombe, 2004; Armour and Yelling, 2004, 2007). This finding emphasizes again the complexity of professional learning and the need to consider not only what teachers should learn, but *how* professional learning should be structured to maximize its effectiveness. Although mindful of Guskey's (1994) warning that no single approach to CPD will meet the learning needs of all teachers at all times, it seems clear that teachers have much (but not everything) to learn from each other. Thus, it can be argued that effective professional development systems will be those that recognize, support and value teachers' attempts to collaborate and to learn informally in communities of practice (Day, 1999; Cordingley et al., 2003, Stoll et al., 2003; Fuller et al., 2005; Armour and Yelling, 2007).

Following Wenger (1998), concepts such as 'professional learning community' (PLC), teacher networks and collaborative professional learning, reverberate throughout the professional development literature (Toole and Louis, 2002, p. 4). All these concepts share a foundation in the social constructivist learning theories of Vygotsky (1978) and Lave and Wenger (1991). Importantly, a PLC approach to CPD suggests that although, at times, teachers will require expert, external knowledge to support their professional development, this form of learning input is not uniquely privileged. Instead, the need for any external input would be established collectively, and the resulting learning shared and developed further with professional colleagues in relevant school contexts. As Lieberman and Miller (2008, p. 206) have argued: 'Professional learning communities . . . hold the promise of transforming teaching and learning for both the educators and students in our schools'.

It is interesting to consider these research findings in the context of the earlier 'Learning Theories' chapter of this book where the authors discuss an 'organic' approach to learning. They cite the work of Davis et al. (2008, p. 11) who define organic learning as being about a 'vibrant sense of connection among people and between humans and the more-than-human world'. Such an understanding of learning seems to resonate with Lieberman and Miller's (2008) claims that effective PLCs can be transformative for teachers and pupils, and also Hodkinson et al.'s (2008) metaphor of learning as 'becoming':

> . . . learning can change and/or reinforce that which is learned, and can change and/or reinforce the habitus of the learner. In these ways, a person is constantly learning through becoming, and becoming through learning. (p. 41)

Learning as 'becoming' is an interesting metaphor in the context of CPD. There is an increasing body of evidence about both the potential and the challenges of establishing PLCs in physical education. Deglau and O'Sullivan (2006, p. 395) reported the success of a long-term CPD programme for physical education teachers in the USA and, in particular, noted that 'its commitment to providing opportunities for teachers to engage with each other within a community of practice, resulted in many of the teachers forming strong identities as teaching professionals'. Ko et al. (2006) also argued that in order to be effective, physical education CPD should be situated and grounded in teachers' practices and O'Sullivan (2007, p. 6) reported that 'when teachers collaborate in such communities they are more willing to take risks, reflect on their failures and share successful programmes and practices'. Yet, as Patton and Griffin (2008) remind us teachers, as individuals, learn in very different ways and establishing collaboration to the level required for effective and sustained learning can be challenging. Similarly, in England, Armour and Duncombe (2004) found that the teachers of primary physical education struggled to learn collaboratively, particularly where a school failed to offer enabling professional learning structures. O'Sullivan (2007) also urged caution, commenting that attempts to introduce, develop and sustain communities of practice resulted in numerous challenges, in particular finding ways to inspire deep and critical discussions amongst the teachers involved. Keay's (2006) research also pointed to difficulties in making the theory of PLCs work in practice. Importantly, these research findings remind us that no single form of professional learning can be viewed as a panacea. It also seems clear that bringing about significant change in CPD must involve not only teachers and schools, but also all those who might reasonably claim to be part of the wider physical education learning community.

Reflection

1. Search for local examples of professional development activities designed for physical education teachers. Try to find out as much as possible about the aims and stated outcomes, learning design, and the intended audience.
2. Undertake an audit of the topics covered in the physical education-CPD available to teachers in your area. Comment on the profile of activities in comparison to the aims of the local or national physical education curriculum. Is anything missing?
3. Consider the implications of viewing learning as 'becoming' for the establishment of effective PLCs with physical education teachers.

The Physical Education Professional Learning Community

I believe that if a course lets you go back to your school and try things, record them, and then go back again and talk about what you've done . . . that would make me learn.

(Primary school teacher from England commenting on teacher learning in the national physical education CPD programme)

We [delegate teachers] discussed the possibility of a follow-up course in order to take that learning to a higher level. The [CPD provider] was positive and set up a follow-up gymnastics course. But it was not as helpful as we expected it to be.

(Secondary physical education teacher from England commenting on the need for learning progression in the national CPD programme)

Physical education teachers work in schools and directly with pupils. We argue, however, that a physical education PLC must also include CPD providers, initial teacher education lecturers, researchers, inspectors/advisors and policy makers. All of these groups have a key role to play in supporting teachers to do their work, and so all are implicated in teachers' professional learning. For example, Stein et al. (1999) suggested that the needs of CPD providers have been neglected, and they argue that what is needed is nothing less than a transformation in their practices. They identified a range of new skills required by CPD providers including being able to develop self-sustaining learning communities in schools, basing teacher development on theories of teacher learning; and understanding better the importance and relevance of individual school contexts. In addition, these researchers emphasize the argument that in order to be considered as professionals, professional developers must take greater responsibility for the impact of their development activities on both teachers' and pupils' learning. We would like to argue that physical education researchers, too, could usefully consider how their research supports teachers' professional learning; including addressing questions about the relevance of the topics they investigate, the ways in which research quality is guaranteed, and the mechanisms that are in place to facilitate effective communication of research. These arguments are not intended to be critical of existing research, researchers or CPD providers, rather they suggest that working more explicitly within a physical education PLC could lead to stronger career-long support for teachers and better learning outcomes for pupils. It is also important to remember, that the physical education PLC is intimately connected to a number of other relevant professional and knowledge communities. As Grossman and McDonald (2008, p. 199) argue there is a need for all groups in education to look beyond immediate communities and 'to look over their backyards to see and learn from what their neighbours are doing'. For example, in the case of physical education, the extended professional community would span different subject communities, elements from sport and coaching and relevant health communities.

What underpins much of the discussion in this chapter is a need for teachers' professional development to be rooted in understandings of the complexities of learning in general, and teacher learning in particular. This would appear to be a logical, albeit not a straightforward proposition. Although some examples of learning theory have been provided in this chapter, and core theories are presented in other chapters on learning theories, there are many other ways to view learning. As Colley et al. (2003) have pointed out, learning is a vast concept and each learning theory tends to view effective learning differently. One way forward, however, would be to accept Claxton's (2007) suggestion that education ought to be about building *learning capacity* in pupils, and then apply the same proposition to teachers and their career-long professional learning. Thus, following Dewey's (1958) theory on learning as the continuing of experience, each professional development activity in the physical education community of practice would be designed to increase teachers' capacity for future learning. Most importantly, perhaps, traditional forms of CPD tend to locate teachers as passive and dependent in the professional learning process. The first task of an invigorated physical education PLC, therefore, should be to empower teachers to be active in their own professional development by encouraging them to demand the support they need in the interests of their pupils (Armour, 2006; Armour and Yelling, 2007). In other words, if we in the physical education profession want to claim that we are indeed deserving of our designation as a profession, then we need to be able to demonstrate that teachers who learn are at the core of our endeavours. More specifically, we should be able to demonstrate that by drawing upon the most current knowledge available in all relevant fields, physical education teachers are striving continuously to improve their abilities to diagnose and meet the learning needs of their clients; that is, all the children and young people they exist to serve. That, in short, is our rationale for placing teachers as learners at the heart of the professional identity of the physical education profession.

Learning More

You will find the following resources helpful in your quest to become a career-long learning professional in physical education: Armour and Yelling (2007) focus on the CPD experiences of physical education teachers, revealing the value they place on learning with and from each other; Lieberman and Miller (2008) explore in more detail the potential of establishing professional learning communities; Day (2004) takes a realistic approach to understanding teachers as human beings who are passionate about learning; and Hodkinson et al. (2008) argue for a holistic approach to learning, conceptualizing it as a process of 'becoming'.

References

Armour, K.M. (2006) Physical education teachers as career-long learners: a compelling research agenda, *Physical Education and Sport Pedagogy*, 11(3), pp. 203–208.

Armour, K.M. and Duncombe, R. (2004) Teachers' continuing professional development in primary physical education: lessons from present and past to inform the future, *Physical Education and Sport Pedagogy*, 9(1), pp. 3–22.

Armour, K.M. and Makopoulou, K. (2008) *Independent Evaluation of the National PE-CPD Programme – Final report.* Loughborough University.

Armour, K.M. and Yelling, M.R. (2004) Professional development and professional learning: bridging the gap for experienced physical education teachers, *European Physical Education Review,* 10(1), pp. 71–94.

—(2007) Effective professional development for physical education teachers: the role of informal, collaborative learning, *Journal of Teaching in Physical Education*, 26(2), pp. 177–200.

Borko, H. (2004) Professional development and teacher learning: mapping the terrain, *Educational Researcher*, 33(8), pp. 3–15.

Brunetti, G.J. (1998) Teacher education: a look at its future, *Teacher Education Quarterly, Fall*, pp. 59–64.

Claxton, G. (2007) Expanding young people's capacity to learn, *British Journal of Educational Studies*, 55(2), pp. 115–134.

Cochran Smith, M. (2005) The new teacher education: for better or worse, *Educational Researcher*, 34(7), pp. 3–17.

Colley, H., Hodkinson, P. and Malcom, J. (2003) *Informality and Formality in Learning: A Report for the Learning and Skills Research Centre*. London: Learning and Skills Research Centre.

Cordingley, P., Bell, M., Rundell, B. and Evans, D. (2003) The impact of collaborative CPD on classroom teaching and learning. In *Research Evidence in Education Library*. London: EPPI-Centre, Social Science Research Unit, Institute of Education, University of London.

Cothran, D.J., McCaughtry, N., Hodges, P.K. and Martin, J. (2006) Top-down public health curricular change: the experience of physical education teachers in the United States, *Journal of In-service Education*, 32(4), pp. 533–547.

Craft, A. (2000) *Continuing Professional Development: A Practical Guide for Teachers and Schools*. Second edition. London: Routledge.

Davis, B., Sumara, D. and Luce-Kapler, R. (2008) *Engaging Minds: Changing Teaching in Complex Times*. Second edition. New York: Routledge.

Day, C. (1999) *Developing Teachers: The Challenges of Lifelong Learning*. London: Falmer Press.

—(2004) *A Passion for Teaching*. London: Routledge Falmer.

Day, C. and Sachs, J. (2004) Professionalism, performativity and empowerement: discourses in the politics, policies and purposes of CPD (pp. 3–32). In C. Day and J. Sachs (eds) *International Handbook on the Continuing Professional Development of Teachers*. Milton Keynes: Open University Press.

Deglau, D. and O'Sullivan, M. (2006) The effects of a long-term professional development programme on the beliefs and practices of experiences teachers, *Journal of Teaching in Physical Education*, 25, pp. 379–396.

Dewey, J. (1958) *Experience and Education*. New York, Macmillan.

DfEE (2001) *Learning and Teaching: A Strategy for Professional Development*. Nottingham: DfEE publications.

Elmore, F.R. (2002) *Bridging the Gap between Standards and Achievement: The Imperative for Professional Development in Education*. Accessed at: www.shankerinstitute.org/Downloads/Bridging_Gap.pdf.

Etzioni, A. (1969) *The Semi-Professions and Their Organisation*. New York: Free Press.

Falk, B. (2001) Professional learning through assessment (pp. 118–140). In A. Lieberman and L. Miller (eds), *Teachers Caught in the Action. Professional Development that Matters*. New York: Teachers College Press.

Fuller, A., Hodkinson, H., Hodkinson, P. and Unwin, L. (2005) Learning as peripheral participation in communities of practice: a reassessment of key concepts in workplace learning, *British Educational Research Journal*, 31(1), pp. 49–68.

Garet, S.M., Porter, C.A., Desimone, L., Birman, B.F. and Yoon, K.S. (2001) What makes professional development effective? Results from a national sample of teachers, *American Educational Research Journal*, 38(4), pp. 915–945.

Grossman, P. and McDonald, M. (2008) Back to the future: directions for research in teaching and teacher education, *American Educational Research Journal*, 45(1), pp. 184–205.

Guskey, T.R. (1994) Results-oriented professional development: in search of an optimal mix of effective practices, *Journal of Staff Development*, 15, pp. 42–50.

—(2000) *Evaluating Professional Development*. Thousand Oaks, CA: Corwin Press.

—(2002) Professional development and teacher change, *Teachers and Teaching: Theory and Practice*, 8(3–4), pp. 381–391.

Hargreaves, L., Cunningham, M., Hansen, A., McIntyre, D., Oliver, C. and Pell, T. (2007) *The Status of Teachers and the Teaching Profession in England: Views from Inside and Outside the Profession*. Final Report of the Teacher Status Project. London: DfES.

Helsby, G., Knight, P., McCulloch, G., Saunders, M. and Warburton, T. (1997) *'Professionalism in Crisis': A Report to Participants on the Professional Cultures of Teachers Research Project.* Lancaster: Lancaster University.

Hodkinson, P., Biesta, G. and James, D. (2008) Understanding learning culturally: overcoming the dualism between social and individual views of learning, *Vocations and Learning,* 1, pp. 27–47.

Huberman, M. (1983) Recipes for busy kitchens, *Knowledge: Creation, Diffusion, Utilization,* 4(4), pp. 478–510.

James, M., McCormick, R., Black, P., Carmichael, P., Drummond, M., Fox, A., MacBeath, J., Marshall, B., Pedder, D., Procter, R., Swaffield, S., Swann, J. and Wiliam D. (2007) *Improving Learning How To learn: Classrooms, Schools and Networks.* London: Routledge.

Keay, J. (2006) Developing the physical education profession: new teachers learning within a subject-based community, *Physical Education and Sport Pedagogy,* 10(2), pp. 139–157.

Ko, B., Wallhead, T. and Ward, P. (2006) Professional development workshops – 'what do teachers learn and use?' *Journal of Teaching in Physical Education,* 25, pp. 367–412.

Lave, J. and Wenger, E. (1991) *Situated Learning: Legitimate Peripheral Participation.* Cambridge: Cambridge University Press.

Lieberman, A. and Miller, L. (eds) (2008) *Teachers in Professional Communities.* New York: Teachers College.

Loughran, J. and Gunstone, R. (1997) Professional development in residence: developing reflection on science teaching and learning, *Journal of Education for Teaching,* 23(2), pp. 159–178.

Makopoulou, K. and Armour, K.M. (2006) Evaluating the National PE-CPD Programme in England: evidence from schools and teachers. Paper presented at the British Educational Research Association Conference, University of Warwick, England, 6–9 September 2006.

Muijs, D. and Lindsay, G. (2008) Where are we at? An empirical study of levels and methods of evaluating continuing professional development, *British Educational Research Journal,* 34(2), pp. 195–212.

O'Sullivan, M. (2007) Creating and sustaining communities of practice among physical education professionals. Paper presented at the AIESEP – Lougborough Specialist Seminar on PE-CPD, Loughborough, England, 1–3 September.

Patton, K. and Griffin, L.L. (2008) Experiences and patterns of change in a physical education teacher development project, *Journal of Teaching in Physical Education,* 27, pp. 272–291.

Penuel, W.R., Fishman, B.J., Yamaguchi, R. and Gallagher, L.P. (2007) What makes professional development effective? Strategies that foster curriculum implementation, *American Educational Research Journal,* 44(4), pp. 921–958.

Pluckrose, H. (1987) *What is Happening in Our Primary Schools?* Oxford: Basil Blackwell.

Rees, J.A. (1999). On being a professional. In P. Mason (ed.), *Tomorrow's Pharmacist.* October. (http://www.pharmj.com/students/tp1999/professional.html)

Sato, M., Chung Wei, R. and Darling-Hammond, L. (2008) Improving teachers' assessment practices through professional development: the case of national board certification, *American Educational Research Journal,* 45(3), pp. 669–700.

Schon, D. (1971) *Beyond the Stable State.* London: Temple Smith.

Shulman, L. (2000) From Minsk To Pinsk: why a scholarship of teaching and learning? *Journal of Scholarship of Teaching and Learning,* 1, pp. 48–53.

Smith, A., and Reading, M. (2001) Reviewing performance management – impact and implications. Paper presented at the British Educational Research Association Annual Conference, University of Leeds.

Sparks, D. (2002) *Designing Powerful Professional Development for Teachers and Principals.* Oxford, OH: NSDC.

Stein, M.K., Smith, M.S. and Silver, E.A. (1999) The development of professional developers: learning to assist teachers in new settings in new ways, *Harvard Educational Review,* 69(3), pp. 237–269.

Stoll, L., Bolam, R., McMahon, A., Wallace, M., Thomas, S., Hawkey, K. and Smith, M.S. (2003) Creating and sustaining effective professional learning communities. Paper presented at the Sixteenth International Congress for School Effectiveness and Improvement, Sydney, Australia, 5–8 January 2003.

Toole, J.C. and Louis, K.S. (2002) The role of professional learning communities in international education. In K. Leithwood and P. Hallinger (eds), *Second International Handbook of Educational Leadership and Administration.* Dordrecht: Kluwer.

Vygotsky, L.S. (1978) *Mind in Society: The Development of Higher Psychological Processes* (trans. M. Cole). London: Harvard University Press.

Wayne, A.J., Suk Yoon, K., Zhu, P., Cronen, S., and Garet, M.S. (2008) Experimenting with teacher professional development: motives and methods, *Educational Researcher,* 37(8), pp. 469–479.

Wenger, E. (1998) *Communities of Practice: Learning, Meaning and Identity.* Cambridge: Cambridge University Press.

West Ed (2002) *Teachers Who Learn, Kids Who Achieve.* San Francisco, CA: West Ed.

5 Teaching as Professional Inquiry

Mary O'Sullivan, Deborah Tannehill and Carmel Hinchion

Chapter Outline

In your professional lives you will enact who you are as a teacher and what you value as education. Sometimes you will act in contradiction to your beliefs and values and will be what McNiff and Whitehead (2005) call 'living contradictions'. As a human being in the teaching profession you will be on a journey experiencing many people, contexts and situations. To understand these experiences you will need to take time to consider them and be thoughtful about them. This commitment to learning from your experiences requires a professional stance of enquiry where you think about and question what you do as a teacher and why you do it.

The focus of this professional enquiry has many interconnecting layers:

- Reflecting on self and self as teacher
- Reflecting on the teaching contexts in your experience
- Reflecting on your students and their learning
- Reflecting on the teaching profession

Understandings of Reflective Practice

The concept of reflective practice has gained a huge following among education and health care professionals in recent decades. It was first made popular by Donald Schon (1983) who described how the complexities of the work of teachers, lawyers, doctors and nurses, among other professionals, requires skilful professional practice and sophisticated professional judgements. This requires a capacity by the teacher to reflect on the circumstances of their teaching. As a teacher you will decide a plan of work to achieve the objectives you have set for your students. As you and they proceed with lessons you will reflect on what the students are learning and if changes are needed to ensure they have a positive and high quality learning experience.

This approach requires an openness to new ideas and development of problem-solving skills to handle the complex teaching situations you will face as a new teacher. In preparing to be a teacher, and during your working life as a teacher, you will grow in understanding yourself as a person and as a teacher. You will develop greater appreciation for, and better understandings of, the students you will teach, the learning environments in which you will work including the ethos of the school, the values of the community and role of parents in the education of their children.

Mirror as a metaphor for reflection

The mirror image is a useful metaphor to explain the process of reflection. When you look in a mirror you can see yourself reflected back. If you take time you can check if you are happy with aspects of yourself. The mirror offers you a perspective and affords you the opportunity to make evaluations and consider changes.

The mirror metaphor can help you to think about your teaching also. When you stop and look in the 'mirror' after having taught a class what do you see? What did you do in the class? What were you thinking and feeling? What were your students doing? Were your practices effective? Are there changes you need to make? How will you make them?

However, reflection does not just happen. It is a habit of mind you develop throughout your life. For example, how would you apply the concept of reflection to the playing of a soccer match? What would be the purpose of this reflection? When would you reflect? How would you reflect? Are there different types of reflection required? What frame of mind do you need to reflect? What questions would you ask? What might be the outcome of this questioning? When and how do actions play a part in reflection?

If you have taken time to consider the last paragraph and attempted to answer the questions you have been engaged in the process of reflection. Taking time to reflect can help you to observe, gain perspective, make decisions, be critical, act in a particular way, challenge beliefs and values, and ultimately to better understand your circumstances. In learning to teach this process of reflection can be one of the ways to facilitate your development as a teacher and is central to your professional integrity.

Professional Enquiry and Reflective Pedagogies

This section provides you with a set of pedagogies to develop different aspects of reflective practice. They are presented thematically building on the notion that reflection can serve numerous purposes. Different pedagogical tools might be better suited to refining certain understandings of the interconnecting aspects of the teacher, teaching, students and learning.

Reflections on Self

Autobiography

Teacher behaviour is critical within the teaching and learning process. This suggests that examining what you do and how you think are key to understanding why classrooms operate as they do, and how they might be changed. Bullough and Gitlin (2001) propose that writing about life experiences (i.e. teacher autobiography) is a means for a novice teacher to examine personal beliefs and assumptions and from that to design strategies to alter these beliefs thus taking responsibility for future actions and behaviours as a teacher.

Berk (1980, p. 90) describes an autobiography as a 'formative history of an individual's life experience' which includes experiences, individual responses to those experiences, and links what an individual comes to believe and value in relation to what has happened in their lives. The process of recording that account may be done through a variety of methods from writing or drawing to a collection of artefacts as evidence.

The educational timeline and autobiography assignment (Appendix A) is a means for you to come to know who you are and what you believe about teaching and learning. The resulting life story may be kept confidential or shared. Syrjala and Estola (cited in Bullough and Gitlin, 2001) suggest that 'while telling a story we reassess our own lives, and while listening to other people tell stories, we acquire ingredients for our own growth'. This implies that sharing life stories may provide insight for changing practice through developing perspectives on the teaching and learning process.

Another way to reflect on your autobiography and growth as a teacher is through imaging. Images are pictures that form in your mind. If you take time to explore them you become more aware of the thoughts, feelings, values, beliefs and assumptions that underpin these visual representations. Images can capture that sense of an experience which can sometimes be elusive to words. Connelly and Clandinin (1988) stated that 'the pictures we create in our minds are part of us and have emotional dimensions'.

Creating a collage of your developing identity may give you scope to 'picture' the many parts involved in your development as a teacher. The word 'collage' has its roots in the French word 'coller', to glue. However, according to McDermott (2002), a collage is not just a glued set of images but an initiation of a dialogue with self and readers. In this dialogue a collage helps you to 'see' in a dimension where understandings of reality take on a different perspective. It is interesting for you to consider what you might include in your collage and also notice what you do not include (see Appendix B).

Peer dialoguing

During your pre-service studies you will interact with peers, lecturers, tutors and school mentors. These interactions offer many opportunities for learning. Your peer group can afford you a special context for '*learning through dialogue*'. Dialogue is a process which involves learning by listening to, and speaking with, others. According to Alexander (2006) it involves 'the ability to question, listen, reflect, reason, explain, speculate and explore ideas' and requires 'a willingness and skill to engage with minds, ideas and ways of thinking other than our own' (2006, p. 5).

The following two peer dialogue pedagogies will help you to develop this openness of mind and willingness to share:

Working with a critical friend
A critical friend is a colleague you trust and who will help you to learn by being honest and supportive. Being 'critical' does not mean being negative but being constructive with feedback so that you become aware of your strengths and the areas where improvement is needed.

To get the most from this learning partnership it is helpful to outline the nature of the feedback you require. It will be advisable for both of you to meet in advance of the class, discuss your concerns about teaching, and identify the type of information to be collected through observation that will provide you with the most assistance. Appendix C provides a template for a guided peer review to assist you in this process.

Dialoguing reflective journals
A reflective journal is a medium through which you can record your thoughts and feelings about your professional development. It can take many shapes (written, visual, digital, hypertext, mixed media and other creative forms) and you can use it as a type of diary of your learning where you describe and reflect on what is happening to you. An excerpt from Tom's reflective journal is presented here:

Pedagogy Class 05/02/08

'The idea of learning through talking interested me in class today. It relates to the work of Vygotsky which we touched on in first year. I found myself really thinking about this after class. The idea that we learn as a community is fascinating. When I thought about my own learning experiences it became clear that social learning played an essential role in my learning development. Listening to each others' views and writing really helps to broaden my understanding and encourages me to think more deeply about aspects I may not have previously considered [. . .] This is an approach I will definitely keep in mind for my own teaching. Again my mind is filled with questions!'

Sharing excerpts from your reflective journal and talking about insights gained can help you integrate your developing personal and professional self. Paulo Freire (1970, 1974, 1998) has written about the emancipatory possibilities of dialogue to name our world (telling our stories to others) and to transform it to create better and more just practices. We are agents in directing our lives and dialogical practice might prepare us for working in a more democratic way with our students.

Reflection on the Teaching Context

Community mapping

To teach young people you must know them. To know them means to spend time talking with them and learning about what they like, how best they like to learn, and what strengths they bring to the classroom. Young people come from families and communities and making a connection with these aspects of a young person's environment can be important in helping them to see the connection between what you are trying to help them to learn and its role in their lives in school and beyond.

Every school is located in a community which has a history and current resources that can enhance the teaching and learning experiences you provide. Too often, especially in larger towns and cities, the school and the community remain isolated from each other, and teachers don't know the locality well enough to see its value in the learning process. Too often we miss the opportunity to incorporate the locale in enhancing our students' learning and their experience of active lifestyles.

It would be critical, as physical education teachers, to learn about the sport, fitness and recreation programmes and facilities that exist in and near the local community so that you can help students to learn about, and access these amenities and services in non-school time. These resources can be used at various times to support and compliment the physical education programme you have planned. Community mapping is a process that promotes increased interaction between the school and the local environs, engaging teachers and students in systematic information gathering about use of the community in the planning of your teaching and in optimizing the learning of your students.

Simple guidelines to complete a community mapping process are provided in Appendix D.

Reflection on Students and Their Learning

Student shadow

Student shadowing is a means of recording a 'snapshot' of student classroom and life experiences. The purpose of student shadowing is to allow you to get to know what it is like to be a child or youth in today's world and it enables you to better understand how students interpret and respond to school life. Bullough et al. (1992) suggest that teachers come to know their role in the classroom based on students' behaviours and interactions. Shadowing students, observing them in the classroom and with their peers, talking to them and seeking their perceptions, allows you to gain a broader and more realistic view of young people in schools. Information gained from shadowing provides the basis for considering and criticizing school practices. Analysis of student responses is a means of identifying areas of student satisfaction and dissatisfaction and for making comparisons of school experience between students. Most informative for you is shadowing students who are quite unlike you; it prompts you to recall your own life as a student and draw comparisons.

Several strategies are useful in student shadowing; observation and interviews being two of the most critical. When observing your students' participation in physical education lessons you will gain information on how students react to the teacher and their peers, to the activities and learning experiences, and what they learned in the lesson. Observations carried out in a systematic fashion will provide you with insight into what is happening in the name of physical education including the context, the 'feel' of the gymnasium, what the students are like, and how the teacher interacts with and responds to the students. A student interview in addition to spending time during the day with the student(s) and informally interacting, adds another dimension to the student shadow. Appendix E provides guidelines on conducting a student shadow study in your own teaching site.

Action research

Action Research is a way of reflecting on what you do as a practitioner. McNiff and Whitehead (2006, p. 1) suggest that as a practitioner-researcher, 'you are aiming to generate theories about learning and practice, your own and other people's'. They state that action research involves asking a range of questions that set up the processes of thinking necessary for a rigorous and systematic approach to understanding and acting on your teaching. These questions include:

- What is my concern about my practice?
- Why am I concerned?
- How do I gather evidence to show reasons for my concern?
- What do I do about the situation?
- What will I do about it?
- What kind of evidence can show how the situation is unfolding?
- How do I make sure my conclusions are reasonably fair and accurate?
- How do I modify my practice in the light of my evaluation? (McNiff and Whitehead, 2005/2006).

Imagine you are having difficulty with behaviour management in one of your classes. Your observations and written reflections on the lesson note students are continually talking and not paying attention to your instructions. You consider talking to your mentor teacher and with her plan an intervention that will help re-establish your authority. From the literature you may gain insight on how to deal with adolescents who are developing their identities,

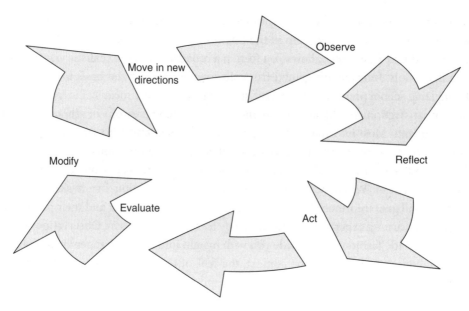

Figure 5.1 Action–reflection cycle (adapted from McNiff and Whitehead, 2006, p. 8).

affiliating with a peer group and questioning authority. In a systematic way you can develop an action plan, implement it and monitor the outcomes. The process has a cyclical pattern of observing, reflecting, acting, evaluating, modifying and moving in a new direction. Figure 5.1 graphically outlines this process.

A key component of this action–reflection cycle is gathering evidence to verify and validate your claims. The data could include a research diary or field notes, interviews, using questionnaires, observation, working with a critical friend, getting feedback from your students, use of video and audio work, online technology, focus groups, social validation groups etc. Your gathered data will help you to reflect on your experience of teaching and act as a touchstone to check against your own perceptions and judgements. It is very important to remember that your data's usefulness lies in its interpretation and consequently its service to the action–reflection cycle.

This type of research gives you a unique opportunity to contribute, even in a small way, to research on teaching and has the important aim of developing knowledge so that you are more empowered in understanding and influencing the practices of your profession.

Reflection on the Teaching Profession

Professional portfolio

A teaching portfolio gives you the opportunity to provide evidence of your teaching practices, reflection on, and interpretation of, those practices for student learning as well as consideration of the role of the teacher in the professional community. You will develop a professional portfolio to highlight that you have developed the skills, knowledge and dispositions reflective of a competent and caring teacher. You will choose the content and evidence to showcase in your portfolio. The evidence you choose to include in the portfolio will come from an array of coursework, learning experiences, and fieldwork.

The 'key' to the evidence selected for the portfolio are your reflections on what you learned from the various experiences, and the impact that learning will have on your teaching and your professional development. As Porter and Cleland (1995, p. 37) noted, 'when students reflect on and interpret their learning experiences paths for personal enquiry about learning emerge'. In this way the portfolio provides a mirror through which you can view, interpret and understand your professional decisions and development as a teacher. Through this process of collecting, analysing and attempting to make meaning of evidence you begin to take responsibility for your own learning. You become aware of your successes as well as the gaps that still exist in your learning, you are able to set goals for future teaching experiences and observe changes that occur over time (Porter and Cleland, 1995).

Lynn et al. (2007) suggest the following types of artefacts (evidence) that might be included in the portfolio:

- *Academic coursework*: Article summaries/critiques, case studies, computer programmes, curriculum plans, essays, goal statements, instructional materials, journals, projects, technology resources, unit plans.
- *Professional development experiences*: Professional organization membership list, honours, Red Cross first aid and CPR certification, WSI certification, photographs, professional reading lists.
- *Field experiences*: Anecdotal records, log books of experiences, evaluations, instructional materials, journals, lesson plans, photographs, technology resources, unit plans, videotapes and audiotapes, student assessments.
- *Work experience*: Evaluations, awards/recognition, resume.
- *Student teaching*: Curriculum plans, long-term planning, evaluations, goals statements, honours, instructional materials, journals, lesson plans, photographs, technology resources, unit plans, videotapes and audiotapes, student assessments, work samples.

The teaching portfolio can be compiled as you navigate your teacher-education programme and include performance-based evidence demonstrating achievement of coursework and teaching experiences. It provides evidence of your achievement in teaching and a detailed description of your understanding of how the evidence relates to effective teaching practice. This allows you to position yourself into how you see the role of the teacher in the teaching profession. Appendix F provides further information about your portfolio.

Final Thoughts

We hope this brief introduction to reflection as professional enquiry has provided you with insight into the critical role reflection plays in the lives of professionals. This should have particular resonance for you as a prospective physical education teacher. As noted previously, reflection is a habit of mind to be cultivated and is central to your growth as a teacher. It develops and refines your teaching knowledge and capacities and ultimately aims to maximize the learning experiences of your students.

It should be apparent from reading this chapter that reflecting on teaching and learning can take place in many ways. You can reflect alone or with colleagues, and in formal and informal settings. You can share your thinking about teaching, learning and schooling in written text, images, or oral conversations with peers, tutors, teachers and lecturers. Discussing your teaching with your students allows you to model reflection as an important part of their learning also.

Typically, your initial reflections as a beginning teacher will focus on concerns for self such as surviving the lesson, managing the students, keeping within the time limits for the class and teaching the content. As you progress in your understanding of students, the curriculum and teaching contexts, your focus will shift to concerns about the appropriateness of the tasks you have chosen for the learning objectives you want the students to achieve. You will become increasingly concerned with how the experiences you are providing your students align with their learning needs and interests and you will concern yourself also with how you assess your learning objectives. Acting on these reflections to improve your teaching is critical as it is in this action that you will improve the quality of your students' experiences.

The strategies and approaches to developing your reflective capabilities allow you to develop and reaffirm your views of education and provide a foundation on which to discuss larger professional issues about the teaching profession, future directions for your profession and appropriateness of the curriculum in contemporary society.

We hope that you have been sufficiently persuaded to try some of these approaches in your teaching. We need creative, and dynamic teachers to critique our current practices, challenge existing values and seek to create and deliver relevant, and meaningful physical activity experiences for the current generation of children and young people. The future of our profession depends on such enquiring professionals.

Learning More

Sources to assist for reflective inquiry on your teaching are available. Some are seminal textbooks on the value of reflection and on educating the reflective practitioner (Schon, 1983, 1987). Others are written for pre-service teachers and provide assignments to reflect on aspects of your development as a teacher (e.g. Bullough and Gitlin, 2001; McDermott, 2002). Still others have been written specifically for those learning to teach physical education (Lynn et al., 2007). Finally there are more general texts detailing particular techniques of professional inquiry such as action research (McNiff and Whitehead, 2005, 2006) and portfolio development (Porter and Cleland, 1995).

References

Alexander, R.J. (2006) *Education as Dialogue: Moral and Pedagogical Choices for a Runaway World.* Hong Kong: Hong Kong Institute of Education in conjunction with Dialogos.

Berk, R. (2003) Arguments for using biography in understanding teacher thinking. In M. Kompf and P. Denicolo (2003) *Teacher Thinking Twenty Years On.* London: Taylor and Francis Publishers.

Bullough, R.V. and Gitlin, A.D. (2001) *Becoming a Student of Teaching: Linking Knowledge Production and Practice.* Second edition. New York: Routledge Falmer.

Bullough, R.V., Knowles, J.G. and Crow, N.A. (1992) *Emerging as a Teacher.* London: Routledge.

Connelly, M.F. and Clandinin, D.J. (1988) *Teachers as Curriculum Planners.* Ontario: Teachers College Press.

Diamond, P. (1991) *Teacher Education as Transformation.* Milton Keynes: Open University.

Freire, P. (1970) *Pedagogy of the Oppressed.* New York: Continuum.

—(1974) *Education for Critical Consciousness.* New York: Continuum.

—(1998) *Pedagogy of Freedom, Ethics, Democracy and Civic Courage,* Lanham, MD: Rowman and Littlefield.

Lynn, S., Costelli, D., Werner, P. and Cone, S. (2007) *Seminar in Physical Education: From Student Teaching to Teaching Students.* Champaign, IL: Human Kinetics.

McDermott, M. (2002) Collaging pre-service teacher identity, *Teacher Education Quarterly,* 29(4), pp. 53–68.

McNiff, J. and Whitehead, J. (2005) *Action Research for Teachers.* London: Fulton Publishers.

—(2006) *All You Need to Know about Action Research.* London: Sage.

Porter, C. and Cleland, J. (1995) *The Portfolio as a Learning Strategy.* Portsmouth, NH: Bounton/Cook Publishers.

Schon, D.A. (1983) *The Reflective Practitioner.* New York: Basic Books.

Syrjala, L. and Estola, E. (1999) Telling and retelling stories as a way to construct teacher's identities and to understand teaching. In Bullough, R.V. and Gitlin, A. (2001) *Becoming a Student of Teaching: Methodologies for Exploring Self and School Context.* Second edition. Madison, AL: Brown and Benchmark.

Part Two
Teaching for Learning

Planning for Learning 6

Tony Macfadyen

It is apparent from the contents page of this book alone that teaching is a multifaceted activity that requires a teacher to make many decisions. As Black and Wiliam (1998, p. 1) point out 'learning is driven by what teachers and pupils do in classrooms. Here, teachers have to manage complicated and demanding situations . . . in order to help [youngsters] to learn now, and to become better learners in the future'. In agreement Holt et al. (2006, p. 103) add 'students will generally learn what you teach' and this is heavily guided by planning. To borrow Goleman's (1995) idea, planning can be viewed as a 'master aptitude' in that it has a capacity to affect many other aspects of teaching and learning, like class management and differentiation. Macfadyen and Bailey (2002) suggest that planning is one of the most significant factors effecting pupil learning since it largely determines what actually happens in the lesson. It is not surprising then that teachers at the beginning of their career can spend considerable time planning (John, 2006) to which Williams (1996, p. 27) has concluded that '. . . for most students, detailed planning is an essential prerequisite for successful teaching'.

There are different sorts of plans for different purposes. Long-term plans help a department prepare schemes of work for the coming year or more, medium-term planning (units of work) is needed for the coming term and short term planning prepares the teacher for the coming lesson. This chapter concentrates, in the main, on lesson planning and examines why planning is important. It goes on to consider the decisions teachers need to make when they plan, and identifies the elements of effective planning that help to promote pupil leaning. Lastly, the chapter offers a distinct way of planning, through a contextual model, to promote pupil learning and offers a critique of the traditional, skill-based, planning philosophy.

Introduction

Common sense allied to research suggests that if pupils are to learn effectively and efficiently, from innovative teaching, appropriate planning is required (DfES, 2002; OfSTED, 2008). The necessity of planning is widely accepted (Kay, 2001) although the format that planning takes is more contested. Theodoulides (2003, p. 16) states that 'an inclusive curriculum does not just happen, it needs to be planned for'. In this light it is somewhat surprising that a review of the literature appears to suggest that few lesson plan formats have been derived empirically, and to complicate matters Johnson (2007, p. 11) has stated that 'much of the planning research fails to examine it as part of a wider process'. However, in one of the most comprehensive reviews of the research that used 85 studies related to planning, instruction and reflection, Hall and Smith (2006) found that 'the act of planning is what often guides lesson focus and content in order to . . . ultimately achieve student learning' (Johnson, 2007 p. 11). Mujis and Reynolds (2005) report effective planning to be associated with positive learning outcomes. In England the QCA (2004, p. 17) has suggested that a clear plan is required 'to make a positive impact on pupils' learning and achievement' and as planning can help sharpen the focus on teaching and learning it contributes to improved standards (DfES, 2002).

Research by John (2006) suggests some trainee teachers find lesson planning difficult to learn, but getting planning right is vitally important because although 'the lesson planning model teachers learn in their methods course are altered and simplified when they become certified teachers . . . the general framework and thought process remain' (Causton-Theoharis et al., 2008, p. 385). Similarly, Bailey and Nunan (1996, p. 15) point out that '. . . while the plans that teachers lay will be transformed in the act of teaching such plans provide a framework and structure for the interactive decisions a teacher must take'.

It appears that planning is rewarded by teacher confidence and improved opportunities for pupils to learn (e.g. see Causton-Theoharis et al., 2008). Bailey and Nunan (1996) report trainee language teachers ranked developing lesson-planning skills as the sixth most important aspect of their development whereas one student summed up the feelings of many in a study by Causton-Theoharis et al. (2008, p. 388) by exclaiming that lesson planning had 'been the single most powerful part of my teacher preparation'. Research by Gammon and Lawrence (2007) found that University sports students' anxiety towards presentations was lessened as they did more preparation. Such experiences have presumably led Durand (1999, p. 452) to state that 'the most important strategy for PE teachers is the lesson plan'. According to John (2006, p. 490),

> whatever approach is taken, the research evidence[of student teachers] points to the fact that the end product – the lesson plan – is often arrived at through a variety of processes, many of which are highly personal, idiosyncratic, and embedded in the subject and classroom context of the topic being planned.

Functions of Planning and Academic Learning Time

Planning provides the backbone to risk assessment and a safe environment which is required for pupil learning. Careful planning provides an opportunity for the teacher to think through the lesson before delivering it. Lessons often generate problems and changing circumstances as they progress so teachers need to be able to think on their feet and maximize unexpected situations. Thus, the more decisions the teacher has been able to think through *before* the lesson begins the better, since their mind will be less cluttered; this is particularly relevant for beginning teachers who have less experience to draw on.

Academic Learning Time (ALT) is often considered to be the connection between teaching and learning; it is the amount of time during which pupils are actively, successfully and productively engaged in learning. More specifically, according to Parker (1989), ALT in physical education (ALT-PE) is that portion of the lesson when pupils are involved with materials that are appropriate to their ability, resulting in high success and low error rates. According to Rink (1996) a task is at an appropriate level of difficulty when the learner can be successful with effort. ALT is of great importance since one of the most consistent research findings is that 'ALT is a strong determinant of academic achievement' (Gettinger and Seibert, 2002, p. 1). However, there is a lot less research on the relationship between ALT and skill learning in physical education where only a few studies examined the relationship between ALT-PE and fundamental motor skill learning. However, given physical education's practical nature that dictates there can be a lot of class management required, planning to ensure high amounts of ALT appears doubly important, not least because further time is lost to pupils changing and getting to the working area. McNeill et al. (2008) have reported that up to 70 per cent of a physical education lesson can be lost to non-ALT which is worrying in light of research by Derri et al. (2007) who found significant relationships between skill acquisition, learning and ALT-PE. The good news is that components of ALT can be seen as manipulable and therefore under the teacher's control. Within the best practice research for increasing ALT, 'proactive planning . . . which includes all steps a teacher takes to be prepared to deliver a lesson' has been identified as one such variable (Gettinger and Seibert, 2002, p. 7).

Reflection

Given the significance of time as a determinant of learning, reflect on what you find most difficult about maximizing ALT-PE. Identify how your planning either helps and/or hinders the time available for pupils to actually engage in the leaning tasks you set them.

Hellison and Templin (1991) found that adequate preparation of equipment can make a great difference to levels of pupil activity and consequently learning and McNeill et al. (2008) found that by changing the planned structure of lessons, trainee teachers could increase the ALT available. Mawer (1995) explains this is probably because teachers who plan their work in physical education (in comparison with those who do not) are able to organize the lessons more carefully, make better use of resources and provide greater variety and better progression of activities. Interestingly, research by Cousineau and Luke (1990) found that teachers' expectations of their pupils in physical education affected the amount of ALT pupils received. High-expectancy pupils had significantly higher ALT-PE measures than middle-expectancy pupils who in turn got more ALT than those pupils for whom teachers only had a low expectation. Clearly such patterns are inequitable, so it is vital all teachers reflect on their practice and consider how planning might ensure a fairer outcome for all.

Reflection

Given the importance of equality in education, list the reasons why you think Cousineau and Luke (1990) obtained the results they did. How will the issues raised in your list affect the way you plan? Can you find any other evidence to support or contradict this research paper?

Planning allows the teacher to visualize the lesson, its activities, its structure and how it is to be delivered. Writing a plan down can give an even clearer idea of how the different elements relate to each other, and to how well they address the objective set. This is of considerable benefit if one considers the wealth of questions that lie implicitly within a plan, such as:

- How do I gain the pupils' attention and interest at the beginning?
- How do I get the lesson off to crisp start but ensure it is safe?
- How shall I arrange the working area and the equipment?

Subject knowledge presents a major source of concern for novice teachers given how wide-ranging physical education is. Many teachers are expected to teach pupils practical skills and how these are applied, through lessons as wide ranging as dance; outdoor activities; swimming and games; also knowledge of health-related activity is usually required and yet some beginning teachers have only a one year training course to learn all this is in. To add further pressure, many students come into physical education from a sports science background which is clearly of limited use.

Lesson planning then, can serve as a valuable aide-memoir where the act of preparing the plan identifies gaps in knowledge and understanding, to prompt further research. This means, crucially, the information is then available to the teacher at the point of delivery to support pupil learning. Moreover, simply having a well-developed understanding of a broad physical education curriculum is insufficient, as the effective teacher must present the curriculum meaningfully. In support, a major research project by the Teaching and Learning Research Programme /Economic and Social Research Council in the UK (TLRP/ESRC, 2007) consistently identified teacher learning as one of the principles underpinning effective teaching and learning. This suggests teachers should regularly examine their own practice and be prepared to change the way they plan, perhaps radically.

Planning can act as a warning in another way. By offering an overview of the lesson ahead, it highlights necessary pre-lesson preparation of resources and possible sources of disturbance. Teachers can think through potential issues that can lead to reduced ALT and many potential problems can be identified *before* the lesson such as spotting possible bottlenecks (that can also cause poor behaviour). For example, time for setting up gymnastic apparatus can be considerably reduced with the aid of a clear plan, especially when displayed for pupils to follow. Gettinger and Seibert (2002) summarize potential problems neatly into:

- Academic (What will I do if pupils struggle to understand the concept?)
- Behavioural (What action will I take if pupils are off task?)
- Administrative (What shall I do with 'non-doers')

Plans also provide a useful record of the teaching and the intended learning that has taken place. Planning is a relatively simple, concrete, means of showing that adequate care and attention has been taken of pupils' learning. There are many times when it is important to have written evidence of work carried out, including a basis from which later work can be developed.

Planning Decisions

In planning, the teacher considers a number of related issues that determine the character of the lessons. One way of the conceptualizing this is as a series of variables relating to the content, the organization and the presentation of the lesson ('COP') (see Macfadyen and Bailey, 2002). Each relates to a different aspect of the lesson, but they are inextricably linked together (see Figure 6.1). By making decisions about the different elements, both for the whole class and for individual pupils, the teacher can create structure which is a key element of a good lesson plan (DfES, 2002). Thinking teaching through in this way can also help reduce anxiety and uncertainty that are natural responses during the early phase of a teacher's career.

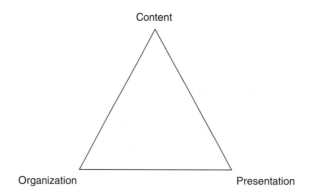

Figure 6.1 The main variables in planning physical education lessons.

Content refers to the identification of knowledge, understanding, attitudes and skills that the teacher aims to develop so it is sensible to start with this variable. In planning for content, the teacher is answering a series of fundamental questions such as:

- What do I want to achieve by the end of the lesson?
- What activities will facilitate success of these objectives?
- How do I progress from one objective to the next?
- How quickly might pupils progress through the activities?
- Are there any particular safety issues that need stating?

Organization refers to the social context of the teaching. Planning for organization ranges from relatively broad issues related to the character of pupil interaction: co-operative, competitive, individualistic, to more specific questions of the size of groups and the arrangement of pupils around the gym. As the teacher considers organizational variables, a series of questions needs to be answered such as:

- How long should the warm up and first practice last for?
- Should the pupils be grouped or work individually?
- If in groups select randomly or by ability?
- What are the different roles that pupils need to take?
- Where will pupils perform and where will the evaluators observe from?

Presentation refers to the way in which the curriculum is taught to the pupils and the best ways of presenting the relevant information to the group. Research suggests effective teaching and learning requires the teacher to 'scaffold' learning, so planned activities should 'support learners as they move forwards, not just intellectually, but also socially and emotionally, so that once these supports are removed, the learning is secure' (TLRP/ESRC, 2007, p. 15). This seems particularly pertinent in physical education, in many countries, where there is a high dropout rate from sport/physical activity when students leave school. The teacher will need to consider *how* pupils will be expected to show understanding of learning, and the most appropriate equipment for the activities. Typical examples of issues might include:

- How will I present the lesson's Intended Learning Objectives?
- How will I expect the pupils to respond, or give evidence that they have understood the concepts or acquired the skills?
- What equipment is most appropriate to support this activity?
- Who will demonstrate and when?

Planning for Learning

Bailey (2001) suggests that where units of work are prepared to a greater depth, pressure on lesson plans is alleviated. Nevertheless, planning for learning in the short term still requires a great deal of thought, especially for inexperienced teachers. Lesson plans provide far more detail about specific activities, short-term goals and teaching strategies. In this respect, then, they form a safety net for the teacher working with a particular class on a particular day.

It is possible to view lesson planning involving four major elements (Kyriacou, 1991):

- Deciding educational objectives
- Selecting and scripting the lesson
- Preparing the props to be used
- Monitoring and assessing pupils' progress.

Deciding and writing educational objectives

It is relatively easy for teachers to build up a collection of enjoyable and worthwhile activities for their physical education lessons. It is more difficult to use these tasks to develop pupils' skills and understanding that make sense to pupils. It is therefore important to plan not only clear lesson objectives, but to provide pupils with '. . . the broad purpose of the lesson, which may directly refer to longer-term objectives and how the lesson links to other lessons' (DfES, 2002, p. 61).

The objectives of a lesson highlight the knowledge, understanding, skills or attitudes the teacher expects the pupils to acquire during the lesson. Objectives should refer to the learning or behaviour of pupils, rather than that of the teacher. They should also be reasonable: in order to gain a clear idea of pupils' progress, objectives need to indicate something the teacher expects the pupils to have achieved by the end of the lesson. Therefore, the teacher needs to break up the targets of a unit of work into manageable elements. For example, a rugby unit might have as a main objective the development of pupils' attacking skills which is too broad for a lesson objective. Depending upon the age and previous experience of the pupils, lesson objectives might refer to pupils' application of the off-side rule in offence or the ability to utilize width in attack.

Thus, Intended Learning Outcomes (ILOs) should be specific so the teacher can actually assess pupil progress against them. One helpful way of writing ILOs in this regard is to include a verb, context and quality (Brunel University, 2004). For example, in badminton:

Verb: Pupils will develop the overhead clear

Context: during co-operative singles play on half-court,

Quality: showing transfer of weight forward into the shot and striking the shuttle at full stretch above the head

Similarly a useful ILO for a lesson plan in invasion games could be: 'Pupils will select and apply a range of passes, in small sided competitive games, demonstrating the importance of penetration in attack'.

The work of Black and Wiliam (1998) has been at the forefront of making the case for stating ILOs at the start of lessons and there is evidence to support their claims. In short, clear ILOs show the pupils what they will be learning and what is expected of them. It is suggested that without planning from objectives, teaching is likely to be less focused and learning more difficult to assess. However, this is only one view, and it needs to be recognized that not everyone believes in its effectiveness. Ainley (2006, p. 23), for example, suggests that 'if teachers plan from objectives, the tasks they set are likely to be unrewarding and . . . impoverished [whereas] if teaching is planned around engaging tasks the pupils' activity may be far richer'. However, Swann (1999; 2003) has launched one of the fiercest and most credible attacks on objectives-based planning detailing ten specific criticisms: 'The objectives model is particularly flawed when it is applied to learning – not least because of its failure to address the open ended nature of human endeavour. Only the most trivial and basic learning can be planned in detail and predicted with accuracy (1999, p. 59). The thrust of the argument is that planning which adheres to an objectives based model incorporates specific flaws, particularly in complex situations (like the physical education setting). Swann suggests a problem-based method instead as it avoids the problems of the objectives model that include:

- a tendency to encourage a blinkered view of what will be possible and successful in practice;
- implementation is prioritized over the issue of to what extent the objectives are worthwhile in the first place; and
- reduces the expression of contention/disagreement and promotes mediocrity (1999, pp. 58–59).

Reflection

Consider what you do at present regarding planning with or without ILOs; think about the strengths and weaknesses you have found to placing ILOs at the start of a lesson for the class. How might the above arguments affect what you do?

Selecting and scripting the lesson

Macfadyen and Bailey (2002) suggest that although physical education lessons necessarily involve physical activity, activity itself is not enough to justify the subject's position in the curriculum, otherwise it could be argued that what is going on is physical recreation and that is appropriate for non-curriculum time. Simply keeping pupils occupied with enjoyable games, it can be claimed, fails to fulfil the educative role of the subject, which demands that pupils learn something. A central aspect of this process is breaking up a larger theme into distinct parts, and designing a progression through them so that they make coherent and intellectual sense to the pupils learning them.

Here the 'r' principle of planning (Macfadyen, 2009) may be helpful as it suggests a lesson plan should have coherence between the different planned elements of the lesson (across the plan) and progression through the lesson (down the plan) so work becomes more difficult as the lesson develops. Figure 6.2 below highlights the 'r' rule with suggestions for effective lesson planning.

In terms of continuity, for example, if the whole class learning is centred on evaluating and improving each others' work, within the teaching styles column the teacher could engage pupils in the reciprocal style as this helps to fulfil the planned objective. That is, the planned teaching style complements the lesson's ILOs. Here, utilizing a 'telling' (direct) style when discovery learning is planned for is counter-intuitive and therefore produces a tension between the two factors which is unhelpful to continuity. However, in a different situation: the safety of throwing events in athletics, planning to use a more didactic style is logical. Furthermore, including Learning Points that support pupils' communication/leadership skills, needed for teaching a partner, will again enhance continuity between the different elements of the plan.

In terms of progression, it stands to reason that pupils may be working on things that are more difficult towards the end of the lesson than at the start and whole class learning activities can and should reflect this. For example, in gymnastics, pupils may begin by working out a routine, of simpler skills, on the floor alone, and progress to include more complex skills on/over benches and tables by the end. Nevertheless, some pupils will be ready for the more advanced work sooner so differentiation by pace, for example, can be planned to match this need. In this way the different parts of the lesson plan add to each other to facilitate pupil learning.

Time	ILOs	Whole class learning activities	Differentiated learning activities	Learning points	Organization of pupils, equipment and resources	Teaching styles and strategies
Start	Should be realistic in number for the time available	These must support the ILOs to promote learning	Consider which differentiation strategies might complement the whole class learning most effectively	Keep relevant to the ILOs.	Important to support the time column	Plan so that the teaching style promotes the intended learning and does not detract from it
Allow enough time for: (i) pupils to explore the learning activities for deep learning; (ii) for assessment opportunities		Less challenging, but appropriate activity, at first		Put in only what you could meaningfully say to a pupil to support their learning (or questions to prompt learning)		
Try to plan activities that follow fluently on from the previous one to save time	These would usually be linked and will build on each other	Each activity then builds on what has gone on before	Think creatively to cater for all abilities / experiences but try to ensure differentiation strategies spur off naturally from the whole class learning activity to cater for	Bullet points can state what the pupils will learn from each activity; 'match up' next to each section which key point(s) you want to get across so you plan to feed points in gradually across the lesson.	Use diagrams where helpful	Continuity
Check your timings so that ALT-PE heavily outweighs organizational requirements	e.g. ILO 1: Pupils work on acquiring a skill	Try not to use too many different activities so the class can concentrate on learning and not coping with change.	• Talented • More able • Pupils at expected level • Less able / experienced		Utilize this column to ensure organization and management issues do not leak into the Learning points column which should be 'clutter'-free	Different approaches are likely to be appropriate at different points in the lesson: look carefully at the ILO and what you are trying to achieve
Be realistic with how longs things will take; do not try to 'cheat' the clock and hence pupil learning	ILO 2: Pupils learn to select and apply the skill	Focus on two or so areas and develop them in different ways so pupils can really engage with the work.				
Progression		More challenging activities stretch the pupils and test out their knowledge, skill or understanding from earlier parts of the lesson	Try to plan for a variety of differentiation strategies across the lesson to help maintain pupils' interest	Ensure learning points are planned for all ILOs	Plan for a little extra resources/equipment as pupils may think up some unexpected ideas/solutions which may need more than first envisaged	Plan using the full range of the 'teaching spectrum' – using a variety of styles will keep things 'fresh' for teacher and pupil alike
Finish						

Figure 6.2 The 'r' principle of planning for learning in physical education (Macfadyen, 2009).

Depending on the philosophy behind the unit being taught and hence the key aims, the teacher may need to consider certain factors more closely. For example, in the Sport Education model an emphasis on team roles across a season (player, coach, umpire, manager, etc.) may mean the teacher needs to be extra vigilant in planning in this regard to ensure different pupils get a worthwhile, long term, experience from what they are tasked to do. Similarly, in TGfU the emphasis on tactical understanding and cognitive development may mean the teacher pays particular attention in planning to their teaching style and the questions they will ask pupils to achieve understanding and success.

It can be a good idea to 'over-plan', particularly while the teacher is adjusting to a new group, in the sense of having sufficient additional activities planned in case the work is too easy or difficult, or is completed quicker than expected. However, this work can be kept in reserve, in case of need; having pupils rush through work just to complete a lesson plan is poor practice as lesson plans do not need to be strictly adhered to (Durand, 1999). Perhaps the key point, it can be argued, is that it is better to cover less, with high quality and deeper understanding, than to cover more work where pupils achieve only superficial understanding. If pupils need longer on one 'episode' of the lesson than anticipated so be it; uncompleted work can be 'shunted' forward to the next lesson. In England, OfSTED (2005, p. 1) have claimed, with some justification, that trying to fit too much into too short a period of time militates against continuity and progression.

Preparing the props to be used

Physical education often involves the use of a range of equipment; it is essential that these resources are prepared and made available by the teacher before the lesson commences. Bad preparation can result in wasted time and worse still accidents. The first stage in preparing the organization part of a lesson might involve the identification and selection of equipment needed. The teacher should aim to match the equipment to the needs of the pupils: How experienced are the pupils? What size equipment will best suit them? Who has a special need that necessitates adapted resources? The teacher also needs to ensure that there is enough equipment for the class being taught: in most cases, plan for individual and small group work to maximize ALT and physical activity.

Monitoring and assessing pupils' progress

In order to determine whether the lesson has been effective in facilitating pupils' learning, it is vital that the teacher monitors and assesses their performance and progress (see Chapter 8). There are many opportunities to assess pupils in physical education and it is important to plan time for these. Of course, the teacher can, and should, observe pupils' learning as they move through the lesson. However, observation is only one method of assessment and pupils can be highly skilled at concealing difficulties (Pye, 1988), so it may be necessary to plan further strategies to probe knowledge and understanding. Transition phases can be used for pupil discussion or teacher questioning but be realistic in planning how long this can take.

Planning for progression

Progression in pupil learning can be enhanced by looking for links and associations between different lessons and units of work so pupils see the larger picture and, importantly, work is not repeated. In England, OfSTED (2005) found that the planned structure of physical education into short units of work, often taught in discrete areas of activity, militated against continuity and progression. Research from the TLRP/ESRC (2007, p. 14) suggests: 'teaching and learning should engage with the big ideas, key processes, modes of discourse and narratives of subjects so that [pupils] understand what constitutes quality . . '. SCAA (1995, p. 21) calls this 'curriculum coherence', as the teacher aims to present the curriculum as a series of related work, not simply as a loose collection of activities. Unfortunately, as Black and Wiliam (1998, p. 10) state: 'surprisingly, and sadly, many pupils do not have a picture, and appear to have become accustomed to receiving classroom teaching as an arbitrary sequence of exercises with no overarching rationale'.

A useful way of contributing to curriculum coherence is to identify common aspects of shared skills or complimentary knowledge between activities, and to draw upon these similarities to consolidate and broaden understanding. This is important as Hofkins (2007, p. 14) points out 'flexibility of mind – the ability to transfer skills and to think methodically but creatively – will be an increasingly hot intellectual property'. A growing body of evidence exists to support the transfer of learning in this manner (Raab, 2007). A good example is the knowledge and understanding of weight transfer learnt in the over arm throw being used to progress learning in the badminton overhead shots.

Progress in difficulty occurs when pupils are required to perform increasingly complex or challenging tasks. When planning, there are many different ways of making tasks more difficult, including:

- challenging pupils to perform more difficult vaults in gymnastic activities;
- asking pupils to devise their own criteria of success for a dance routine; and
- inviting pupils to develop strategic ideas such as how to outwit various defensive patterns in invasion games.

A lack of planning can mean some pupils are under-challenged (and therefore misbehave through boredom) whilst others are over-challenged, causing anxiety, which can manifest itself in pupils either misbehaving (to save 'face' with peers) or not actively participating at all.

Progress in quality can be seen as pupils exhibit increasingly more sophisticated or successful performance of acquired skills. This can take a number of forms, including:

- better clarity or articulation or shape in gymnastics;
- improved co-ordination in ball skills;
- better poise, grace, and fluency in dance; and
- more refined strokes in swimming.

The key point to consider when planning is *what the learning will look like* so the teacher can both reward success and explain/demonstrate it clearly to others in the class. Simply writing 'differentiation by outcome' in a plan, without explaining or providing detail of how this might happen, is insufficient to support pupil learning. Similarly research indicates that it is important to plan the questions the teacher intends to ask pupils (McNeill, 2008).

Progress in context refers to pupils' ability to integrate actions into increasingly complex situations, such as taking more initiative and responsibility in planning, performing and evaluating tasks. However, research suggests that activities need to be specifically planned if teaching and learning is to be effective (TLRP/ESRC, 2007). For example, in dance, the teacher must decide which teaching style is most suitable to improve pupils' ability to self-assess since research has shown 'that being able to talk about their own learning helps students become better able to manage it, more confident and positive . . .' (ibid., p. 15). Readers are referred to Chapter 8 for more on assessment for learning (AfL).

Other important features of lesson planning

Learning Points

As well as a description of the different activities that pupils will be carrying out, lesson plans need to include explicit Learning Points, which highlight important details related to each Learning Activity.

- What are the key points of a new technique that will 'unlock' pupil success?
- What qualities of movement or technical details will the teacher look for?
- Are there specific words or concepts that need to be introduced?

Questions of this sort, and a plan of *when* to introduce different learning points (so pupils are not over whelmed at any stage), help the teacher ensure that the lesson promotes safe and worthwhile learning rather than just activity. Learning points should be *useful* to the pupil so they need to be couched in terms of what pupils need to do rather than as an outcome. For example 'throw as far as you can' is not a useful learning point as it does not help the pupil succeed (and may well be part of the ILO in some form anyway); what the pupil needs to know is *how* to throw further. In this light, a planned learning point such as 'fling your arm through fast and last' will be more helpful.

Transitions

It is in the periods of transition between one activity and another that valuable time can be lost, and problems of misbehaviour often occur. An instruction to 'get a ball' or 'get into groups of three' can lead to chaos with 12 year olds. At least in the early stages of teaching, these organizational issues need to be carefully planned and should always reflect what is known about the class. Considerable time can be saved by planning a demonstration first, with one group, before bringing the rest of the class in to observe the learning. Additionally, sensitive planning like this avoids placing the individuals in the demonstration under undue pressure and gives them a chance to practice first so the key point should be made more effectively.

Non-participants

Readers may like to consider how many non-doers they have in their classes as this can be a good barometer of how enjoyable their lessons are! Nevertheless, physical education places particular demands upon pupils, and it sometimes happens that individuals are unable to participate because of injury/illness. Sitting in the corner of the gym simply watching others is not a valid option and there is more to the non-doer's role than collecting up cones! Instead, the teacher should plan activities in which non-doers can engage with the learning (sometimes in different ways) but does not involve active participation; non-doers can often be exposed to excellent cross curricular learning opportunities. Figure 6.3 below, offers some suggested activities for non-participants.

- Taking the role of a sports journalist by writing up the lesson or a report on an event to improve literacy (posted onto the school intranet for the class to read)
- Taking the role of a sports commentator to improve verbal communication skills
- Taking the role of a sports summarizer to improve analytical and verbal communication skills
- Taking the role of a judge in gymnastics while others perform their routines; more able pupils can create an assessment sheet for the rest of the class to use in the evaluate and improve section.
- Improving ICT skills by acting as a PE technician; recording performances on a digital camera or camcorder and up loading them to school intranet, or analysing pupils' work using sports specific software.
- Taking the role of a choreographer in dance
- Learning the skills to referee (less able/experienced); umpiring a game
- Learning the skills to coach others; coaching others (more advanced/confident)
- Ask the non-doer to assess (certain) pupils' and to design a new, innovative and enjoyable, activity to develop their learning
- 'Scale down' the learning – if the class is learning to apply spin in tennis, can the non-doer do likewise in table tennis?

Figure 6.3 Some suggested activities for non-participants.

The Structure of a Physical Education Lesson

There are different ways to plan a lesson; one example was offered in Figure 6.2 and a further, relatively simple, example is shown in Figure 6.4. See Kay (2001) for an example of a more detailed and completed lesson plan.

Lesson plan			
Theme/Unit:			
Date/time: Class/No. of pupils:			
Learning objectives:			
1			
2			
Reference to statutory requirements:			
Resources and equipment:			
Safety/Risk assessment:			
Phase/timing	Pupils' activities	Learning points	Assessment
Introduction			
Warm up			
Development activities/ S.S.G			
Cool down			
Plenary			

Figure 6.4 An example of a simple lesson plan.

If one considers some of the key, research-based, principles of promoting learning (see below), it seems sensible to suggest a planning philosophy that can actively promote these factors.

- Pupil motivation and enjoyment
- Quality pupil–teacher interactions
- Challenging pupils to work one step ahead of their current level
- Active engagement of the learner, including the promotion of learners' independence and autonomy, such as through AfL (see TLRP/ESRC, 2007; DCSF, 2008; Hattie, 2008).

Creating context

Macfadyen and Bailey (2002) have noted that lesson planning should not ignore the great amount of skill development that occurs implicitly as a result of a well-chosen game or whole activity. For this reason, there are likely to be many times when the 'skill development' part of a lesson needs to be placed in context to give it authenticity and meaning. In particular, how might the physical education teacher plan tasks in such a way that pupils are likely to engage with the intended knowledge in a meaningful, physically educated, way? Swann (1999, p. 57) suggests that 'when a plan is required to address a problem, the context should be scrutinized before launching in with a solution' and Ainley et al. (2006) have noted the importance of context to motivation. For example, it would seem ridiculous to work on the details of a competent swimmer's strokes before creating the context of that detail (by letting the pupil swim). In games, specific skills often only make sense in relation to the game of which they are a part. Pupils need to understand the game as a whole in order to appreciate how the different skill elements fit together. In football, practicing short, simple, side foot passes within a small group can be both uninspiring and meaningless unless they have come out of an analysis of the pupils' *own* game play (e.g. the importance of accuracy in passing for possession, and the pass and move principle to advance the ball up field). The contextual model helps understanding emerge through authentic activity and aims to inspire pupils' to participate, and keep learning what is intended, rather than have pupils (deviously) doing their own thing or have the teacher face those two age-old questions from pupils who have stopped work, with sagging shoulders, and in dispirited voices ask: 'I don't get it: why are we doing this?' or 'can we play a game now?'.

When someone understands *why* they are doing something it can effect motivation (Weinberg and Gould, 2002) and Papaioannou and Goudas (1999) remind us pupils often ask themselves whether they actually *want* to do a task in physical education even if they can. It is proposed here that the contextual model (see below) is more likely to lead to them answering 'yes, I want to' since the lesson will be both more enjoyable (by letting pupils 'have a go' at, and containing more, games and pupil-centred learning) and more understandable (as pupils will know why they are doing something and where it fits in to the activity/sport;

see Griffin et al., 2005). As Launder (2001, p. xii) notes 'the primary task . . . is to help youngsters become competent and enjoy participating . . .they are then more likely to maintain their involvement in the future . . .'.

The contextual model then draws on the situated cognition research which has pointed to the importance of a sense of purpose for pupils in their education. Kirk (2005) has argued that the transfer of authentic and meaningful player experiences into games situations promotes more complete learning of, and motivation toward, playing games. For these reasons, the contextual model of planning for learning may be most appropriate:

1. A vision for the learning to follow
2. Activity related warm-up
3. 'Have a go': whole/context activity (e.g. small-sided game) – Let pupils play/do the 'whole' (if safe); plus appropriate observation (e.g. is my initial planning appropriate? Where does the lesson need to go?)
4. Skill development as required
5. Context activity (e.g. full stroke in swimming) – pupil and teacher assessment
6. Skill development as required
7. Context activity – pupil and teacher assessment
8. Cool down and Plenary

The model aims to build children's practical skills within an understanding of when and why they are used. By letting pupils 'have a go' the teacher not only 'buys' time to assess the pupils but on most occasions, will 'win' the pupils over to their side since the act of playing a game or actually swimming a few widths, for example, means pupils can 'get it out of their system'. In all likelihood they will then be more responsive to listen to, and work with, the teacher's planned ideas. It is important to remember that pupils have a large part to play in what goes on in their lessons, so a teacher is wise to consider the pupils' perspectives. In the above example (3), (5) and (7) provide an overall picture for meaning; pupils' try out and consider what to do and through (4) and (6) how to do it (e.g. the skill/s required to succeed). Neither aspect is more important than the other and the skills act as the 'vehicle' by which pupils can access learning to the overall aim (e.g. to swim efficiently). The use of numbering here does *not* indicate a mechanical way of planning, but serves to highlight the fluid nature of planning that dips into and out of skill development practices as required and when relevant so pupils are aware of the context (meaning) of their work. John (2006) notes that research on expert teachers suggests they 'seem to have a very general plan for lessons, leaving detailed decision-making to the period prior to starting the lesson *or to various points in the lesson itself*' (John, 2006, p. 489, my emphasis).

In planning this way, the teacher's role is more one of facilitator, offering support and guidance with specific problems or extending a child's repertoires of skills but with the potential to blend in the best of direct (active) teaching (through, for example, utilizing the teacher's pedagogic expertise and formative feedback) which is probably the most efficient way of teaching technique (Siedentop and Tannehill, 2000). Of course, the model needs to be linked to appropriate teaching styles, so a teacher must plan accordingly (e.g. indirect/productive styles; see Macfadyen and Bailey, 2002). It can be argued that given the fluid nature of the contextual model a plenary is particularly important to bring the lesson to a thoughtful and contemplative close. For example paired pupil discussions can usefully involve *all* pupils in reflecting on their learning. Research has highlighted the importance of plenaries to the learning process, and shows that planned plenaries tend to be more effective than spontaneous ones (DfES, 2002).

The teacher and pupils together assess progress and plan future learning from and during the context activity which can be a meaningful way for pupils to receive formative feedback (see Griffin et al., 2005). Thus, if some pupils are already demonstrating competence of the lesson objectives during the early part of the lesson they negotiate a more difficult challenge rather than being 'taught' something they can already do! It is then more likely that pupils will *value* their experience of physical education that Kirk and MacPhail (2002) suggest is important, increasing motivation and the likelihood of further participation.

The interactive nature of the model provides a framework that can apply equally to dissimilar activities but pupils remain at the centre of their own learning to provide a sense of excitement, discovery and enjoyment. The work of Wankel and colleagues (e.g. see Wankel, 1985) and more recently Scanlan et al. (1993) highlights the importance of fun and enjoyment to the sports experience; however, further research is needed.

There is, however, a growing body of research in physical education that would support the contextual model as it suggests planning lessons that are structured around both the psycho-motor and cognitive domains is helpful to pupils' development (e.g. Allison and Thorpe, 1997; Light, 2002; Butler et al., 2003; Metzler, 2005). One of the best known and most researched models is the TGfU approach (Bunker and Thorpe, 1982) which provides an organizing structure to promote greater pupil reflection and self-direction as it moves beyond the learning and applying of technical skills to incorporate cognitive development and the socio-cultural aspects of sport (Holt et al., 2002). TGfU has 'now gained widespread acceptance' according to Light (2005, p. 211) and has been established as '. . . a legitimate conceptual framework for games teaching' (Griffin, 2005, p. 214). However other variations of the model are also being developed (e.g. see Raab, 2007 [SMART model]; Launder, 2001 [Play Practice] and Alexander and Penney, 2005 [Clinic-Game Day]). Readers are referred to Chapter 14 (Theories of Learning) for a detailed account of this related area.

The teaching of such 'blended' planning however is not easy and has been found to be problematic (McNiell, 2008); and see McMorris (1998) for a criticism of TGfU. The contextual model presented here requires the teacher to have very good subject knowledge of the sport/activity concerned, a variety of teaching methods, including effective questioning techniques and be able to *recognize* which skills or principle of play are required should the pupils be unable to reach the learning objective. Research by O'Leary (2008) suggests this is very difficult for the novice teacher and Johnson (2007, p. 11) adds 'the planning literature seems to indicate that experienced teachers' plans are more efficient and relevant to the curriculum and to student learning than those of novice teachers'. It is, therefore, suggested beginning teachers ensure they:

1. have ample opportunity to engage with model lesson plans;
2. work closely with their mentor so their learning of planning is 'scaffolded' through a dialogue with real teaching situations (John, 2006);
3. gain access to expert teachers' knowledge through joint planning;
4. reflect on their planning as part of the post-lesson discussion (see Macfadyen, 2008);
5. access additional training in areas of weak subject knowledge.

With this in mind some common errors in planning and alternative suggestions are outlined in Figure 6.5.

Common planning errors	Alternative/solution
Confused or unspecific ILOs so pupils are not clear on what they are to learn / do	Present material which is meaningful to pupils' stage of development; use ILOs that contain a verb, context and quality and link to the pupils' overall learning for the year/Key Stage ('bigger picture').
Too many ILOs (often caused by too many aims/objectives and too few lessons in a Unit of Work)	Be realistic in what (high quality) learning pupils can attain in one lesson; stick two or so main themes or ideas. Avoid short units of work – plan for pupils to work on an activity over an extended period (e.g. 12–16 hours).
Ongoing assessment not used to set future learning targets (e.g. ILOs not linked from one week to the next)	Teaching should take account of what learners know already in order to plan their next steps. This means building on prior learning so use a simple assessment page in which to record pupils' progress and place behind each plan for easy referral when the next lesson is planned.
Unrealistic timings	Do not try to cheat the clock! Allow adequate time for changing, transitions and demonstrations. Do not try to squash too much into the plan.
Time taken to set up a practice is longer than the learning time pupils have on it	Plan carefully where resources are put for accessibility; try to move logically and smoothly from one activity to the next (e.g. plan for 2's to become 4's and so on).
Expecting miracles!	Do not rush to get through an overcrowded plan; e.g. pupils cannot analyse a performance, prepare their points and feed back to a partner in 3 minutes; 10–15 is more realistic to achieve some quality.
A feverish desire to stick to the plan during the actual lesson despite evidence that things are not working	Teach what you see: if pupils are under challenged with what you have planned, adapt the plan accordingly; e.g. skip past a couple of easier practices straight to something more difficult. If the plan is over challenging in games e.g. 5vs3 is too hard, change to 6vs2.

Figure 6.5 Some common errors in beginning teachers' planning.

The 'Traditional' approach

John (2006, p. 492) notes that it is well recognized that some inexperienced student teachers need 'concrete, even prosaic, models of planning to guide their thinking'. An alternative to the contextual plan exists via the more traditional [technique-led] approach to lesson planning which, due to its simplicity, provides a model for beginning teachers who want to retain more control over the lesson and pupils at the expense of responsiveness and flexibility. The traditional approach has four main parts:

1. Introduction
At the start of the lesson, the teacher needs to

- gain the pupils' attention
- introduce the theme of the day's lesson (ILOs)
- possibly review related work from previous lessons, and
- physically prepare the pupils for movement (warm-up).

2. Skill development
This section of the lesson centres on practising specific skills associated with an activity. In dance, for example, pupils might perform certain dance actions. Bott (1997, p. 30) describes the skill development phase as the most important part of the lesson.

3. Climax
During this section of the lesson pupils have the opportunity to apply the skills they have been developing. This could be a short dance routine, utilizing the various 'moves' practised or an opportunity to practice a skill in a game.

4. Conclusion
During the final phase of the lesson, pupils are both cooled down and calmed down by doing gentle, rhythmic exercise; the key points of the lesson are recapped to reinforce lesson content, perhaps through questioning pupils on their understanding.

Perhaps one of the biggest criticisms of the traditional lesson plan is that many pupils do not always understand the purpose of what they are doing so it can leave them frustrated or confused since they have to wait until the end of the lesson to play a game (the very heart of the activity that is most exciting) and unless the teacher is careful the climax can be squeezed out due to lack of time. Pope (2005, p. 272) suggests a model of this nature creates '... machine-like, mindless and often tedious drills that have little meaning for participants or connection for them to the wider game picture'. Ainley (2006, p. 23), more sympathetically, suggests it is the play paradox that is at the centre of the issue:

> . . . the play paradox recognises an inherent tension in the teaching-learning process. Play can facilitate learning and so there is a desire to incorporate play-like freedom into more formal school based learning, even for older pupils. However, such a strategy transfers control over what is learned away from the teacher to the pupils themselves. This is unsatisfactory if the teacher has an agenda in which certain specific knowledge should be assimilated.

As a teacher it is always useful to empathize with your pupils and ask 'how would I want this lesson taught to me?' A most likely answer is in an enjoyable, engaging and interesting way and critics of the traditional approach posit that it cannot deliver this effectively. For example, upon entering the sports hall pupils are faced by any number of basketball hoops and a box of balls; readymade team mates and opposition players are to hand and there is an ideal space to play in; it might not be unreasonable to think pupils' response would be 'let's play!'. However, instead of being allowed to express this natural desire to play a game (which the contextual model promotes), pupils are made to practise passing in dry, isolated, drills that appear to have little relevance or use to the game they are desperate to play. All the time the baskets are 'calling' to pupils 'shoot, shoot' until temptation swallows them up and they take some shots, only to be met with the teacher's disapproving comment 'What are you doing? Did I say to do that? We are working on passing'. Thus, many beginning teachers find themselves having to deal with disciplinary matters they have created in planning because they have bored pupils into misbehaviour by using under challenging and/or uninteresting drills/practices. This point is well made by Griffin et al. (2005):

> We argue that when students request a game, students take the position that games, as compared to skill practices, are fun! One reason games are more fun is that they have structure and outcomes that give meaning to performance, which could be directly tied to situational interest. Situational interest . . . provides a sense of novelty and challenge, demands exploratory action and high level attention, and generates a feeling of instant enjoyment. (p. 220)

Traditional lesson plans also appear problematic in supporting worthwhile pupil assessment as the teacher is likely to move from a warm-up straight into the first practice without observing the pupils in the context of the activity. As a Teacher Trainer I have witnessed lessons where student teachers dutifully take pupils, stage by stage, through some (decent) skill development practices without first bothering to find out what the pupils can do! Pupils often practise (play!) between lessons so it is advisable to re-assess them, even briefly, at the start of each lesson as 'few people these days believe that children arrive at school as "empty vessels" to be filled with knowledge' (TLRP/ESRC, 2007, p. 15); so the principle of starting where children 'are' and helping them to move on is widely recognized (e.g. Hofkins, 2007).

A criticism of games teaching in the UK is that teachers focus too much on acquiring and developing skills and fail to teach pupils to select and apply those skills in the game situation (OfSTED, 2004). In part this may be due to the over use of a traditional model since it pushes teachers in this direction. Additionally, the teacher may well have lost some of the pupils' interest by the time the game finally comes around so although pupils have been present they are in fact 'mind truant' so they find applying skills to the game more difficult still. The problem is exacerbated if the teacher plans to use a direct (didactic) teaching style so pupils have less responsibility for their learning; it could well have been a combination of these factors that led Docking (1996, p. 27) to note, in England, that 'the high work rate of teachers often stood in sharp contrast to the low work rate of the pupils'.

Reflection

Discuss with your peers/tutor/mentor the strengths and weaknesses of planning via the contextual model compared to the alternative, traditional, method.

Pupils' responses to learning create an ever changing dynamic that means there is uniqueness to teaching physical education classes and planning needs to be able to capture this. This suggests that if improvisation, creativity and spontaneity are to be developed the lesson plan will need to be more flexible and less prescriptive than a linear model posited by a traditional approach. Unless teachers are adaptable in their planning and delivery there is a danger pupil opportunities for self reflection are lost – the exact opposite of engaging pupils in their own learning for which we should be striving. There is support for this type of organic planning (reacting to the uncertainty of classroom interactions by using plans that can respond to pupils' needs and where specific targets emerge from broader objectives through teacher/pupil assessment of an activity). Jones and Vesiland (1996) found that as student teachers gained experience their planning shifted from a tight script to a larger cluster of concerns that included class management, the organization of learning and a need for more flexibility. Causton-Theoharis et al. (2008) have suggested educators need to rethink planning so they are more student-centred, and shape creative and active learning for pupils. These authors go on to claim that in education generally teacher-directed, traditional, instruction has contributed to certain populations of students failing for decades perhaps because pupils' responses are in no way predictable or 'prescribe-able' (Ben-Peretz, 2001).

Conclusion

Planning for learning is a complex area but is an essential feature of effective pupil learning. As the demand on our subject to make a notable contribution to children's education increases, now is an ideal opportunity to rethink our planning philosophy and challenge existing and entrenched practices. To some extent, the idea of the contextual model remains speculative however it is based on the constructivist approach, soundly researched teaching-learning principles and is aligned with the well researched TGfU model. As the knowledge base of effective teaching and learning moves forward so must our planning skills. Kirk and MacPhail (2002) have, quite rightly, argued we need to know more about this area, but in the meantime it is suggested that creative, thought-provoking and flexible plans replace traditional rigidity. This chapter has suggested a number of ideas for developing planning, and it has challenged the idea that planning in physical education needs to involve pupils ploughing through unexciting practices and drills. Perhaps what teachers need to ask themselves most is 'which way of planning will excite, interest, engage and motivate my pupils?'

Learning More

Causton-Theoharis et al. (2008) in a thought provoking article from the USA consider a research project on helping pre-service teachers to reconsider how they plan their lessons to be more inclusive and to improve the learning outcomes for all pupils. It is also useful for considering the constructivist lesson design (for student-centred pedagogy) and the traditional teacher-directed instruction as well as a section that links theory to practice. TLRP/ESRC (2007) is a website providing extensive and useful coverage of a large-scale research project in the UK, across a variety of subjects. It presents ten principles of effective teaching and learning and what really makes a difference in pupil learning. Launder (2001) focuses on teaching game play first instead of technique and skill. It provides both the theoretical basis and the practical plans for achieving an innovative and versatile approach to physical education; it therefore provides a valuable appendage to some of the ideas presented in this chapter. Ainley et al. (2006) explore what they call the planning paradox: whether to plan from objectives or not. It sets out a new way to think about planning and concludes with some guidelines to support the new way of thinking. As the focus of the article is mathematics it widens out the context of this chapter, suggesting that our subject is not alone in facing up to the challenges of this area. Finally, there is a special issue of the journal *Physical Education and Sport Pedagogy* (Volume 10(3) November 2005) containing a series of articles relating to TGfU from an international perspective. It provides an excellent overview of the area, detailing the strong research available, how TGfU has gained widespread acceptance and challenges the technique-led approach to physical education teaching.

References

Ainley, J. Pratt, D. and Hansen, A. (2006) Connecting engagement and focus in pedagogical task design, *British Educational Research Journal*, 32(1), pp. 23–38.

Allison, S. and Thorpe, R. (1997) A comparison of the effectiveness of two approaches to teaching games within physical education. A skill versus a games for understanding approach, *British Journal of Teaching Physical Education*, 28, pp. 9–13.

Alexander, K. and Penney, D. (2005) Teaching under the influence: feeding games for understanding into the sport Education development-refinement cycle, *Physical Education and Sport Pedagogy*, 10(3), pp. 287–301.

Association for Physical Education (2002) *Health Position Paper*. Reading: afPE.

Bailey, K.M. and Nunan, D. (1996) *Voices from the Language Classroom*. New York: Cambridge University Press.

Bailey, R.P. (2001) *Teaching Physical Education*. London: Kogan Page.

Ben-Peretz, M. (2001) The impossible role of teacher educators in a changing world, *Journal of Teacher Education*, 52(1), pp. 48–56.

Black, P. and Wiliam D. (1998) *Inside the Black Box*. London: Kings College.

Bott, J. (1997) Developing lesson plans and units of work. In S. Capel (ed.), *Learning to Teach Physical Education in the Secondary School*. London: Routledge.

Brunel University (2004) Effective Lesson Planning. PGCE Physical Education course material (unpublished).

Bunker, D and Thorpe, R. (1982) A model for the teaching of games in the secondary school, *Bulletin of Physical Education*, 10, pp. 9–16.

Butler, J. Griffin, Lombardo, B.L. and Nastasi, R. (eds) (2000) *Teaching Games for Understanding in Physical Education and Sport*. Reston, VA: NASPE.

Causton-Theoharis, J., Theoharis, G. and Trezek, B. (2008) Teaching pre-service teachers to design inclusive instruction: a lesson planning template, *International Journal of Inclusive Education*, 12(4), pp. 381–399.

Cousineau, W.J. and Luke, M.D. (1990) Relationships between teacher expectations and academic learning time in sixth grade physical education basketball classes, *Journal of Teaching Physical Education*, 9(4), pp. 262–271.

Derri, V., Emmanouilidou, K., Vassiliadou, O. and Olave, E.L. (2007) ALT in PE: is it related to fundamental movement skill acquisition and learning? *International Journal of Sports Science*, 3(3), pp. 12–23.

DCSF (2008) The National Strategies: Secondary – The Framework for English: long, medium and short term planning. http://nationalstrategies.standards.dcsf.gov.uk (accessed: 23 April 2009).

DfES (2002) *Key Stage 3 National Strategy: Training Materials for the Foundation Subjects*. London: DfES Publications.

Docking, J. (1996) *Managing Behaviour in the Classroom*. London: Fulton.

Durand, M. (1999) The teaching task and teaching strategies for physical educators (pp. 437–558). In Y. Vanden Auweele, F. Bakker, S. Biddle, M. Durand and R. Seiler (eds), *Psychology for Physical Educators*. Champaign, IL: Human Kinetics.

Gammon, S. and Lawrence, L. (2007) Csiksztmihalyi's flow theory applied to student learning. LINK: Special edition. www.hlst.heacademy.ac.uk

Gettinger, M. and Seibert, J. (2002) Best practices in increasing academic learning time. www.aea1.k12.ia.us/docs/gettinger.pdf (accessed: 8 April 2009).

Goleman, D. (1995) *Emotional Intelligence*. New York: Bantam Books.

Griffin, L., Brooker, R. and Patton, K. (2005) Working towards legitimacy: two decades of Teaching Games for Understanding, *Physical Education and Sport Pedagogy*, 10(3), pp. 213–224.

Hall, T.J. and Smith, M.A. (2006) Teacher Planning, instruction, and reflection: what we know about teacher cognitive processes, *Quest*, 58, pp. 424–442.

Hattie, J. (2008) *Visible Learning: A Synthesis of over 800 Meta-Analyses Relating to Achievement*. Oxford: Routledge.

Hellison, D.R. and Templin, T.J. (1991) *A Reflective Approach to Teaching Physical Education*. Champaign, IL: Human Kinetics.

Holt, J. Ward, P. and Wallhead, T. (2006) The transfer of learning from play practices to games play in young adult soccer players, *Physical Education and Sport Pedagogy*, 11(2), pp. 101–118.

Hughes, P. (2008) *Principles of Primary Education*. London: Routledge.

John, P. (2006) Lesson planning and the student teacher: rethinking the dominant model, *Journal of Curriculum Studies*, 38(4), pp. 483–498.

Johnson, D.A. (2007) Research works: teacher planning, instruction and reflection, *Journal of Physical Education, Recreation and Dance*, 78(5), p. 11.

Jones, M.G. and Vesiland, E.M. (1996) Putting practice into theory: changes in pre-service teachers' pedagogical knowledge, *American Educational Research Journal*, 33(1), pp. 61–119.

Kay, W. (2001) Lesson planning with the NC physical education, *The Bulletin of Physical Education*, 37(3), pp. 189–204.

Kirk, D. (2005) Future prospects for TGfU. In L.L. Griffin and J.I. Butler (eds), *Teaching Games for Understanding: Theory, Research and Practice*. Champaign, IL: Human Kinetics.

Kirk, D. and MacPhail, A. (2002) Teaching Games for Understanding and situated learning: rethinking the Bunker-Thorpe Model, *Journal of Teaching Physical Education*, 21, pp. 177–192.

Kyriacou, C. (1991) *Essential Teaching Skills*. Hemel Hempstead: Simon and Schuster.

Launder, A.G. (2001) *Play Practice – The Games Approach to Teaching and Coaching Sport*. Champaign, IL: Human Kinetics.

Light, R. (2002) The social nature of games: Australian pre-service primary teachers' first hand experiences of teaching Games for Understanding, *European Physical Education Review*, 8(3), pp. 286–304.

—(2005) An international perspective on Teaching Games for Understanding, *Physical Education and Sport Pedagogy*, 10(3), pp. 211–212.

Macfadyen, T. (2008) The 'REVIEW' framework: improving student teachers' lesson debriefs. Paper presented at British Education Research Association, Herriot Watt University, Edinburgh, 3–6 September 2008.

—(2009) The 'r' principle of planning. PGCE Physical Education, The University of Reading; unpublished.

Macfadyen , T. and Bailey, R. (2002) *Teaching Physical Education 11–18*. London: Continuum.

Mawer, M. (1995) *The Effective Teaching of Physical Education*. London: Longman.

Mujis, D. and Reynolds, D. (2005) *Effective Teaching – Evidence and Practice*. London: Sage.

McMorris, T. (1998) Teaching Games for Understanding: its contributions to the knowledge of skill acquisition from a motor learning perspective, *European Journal of Physical Education*, 3, pp. 65–74.

McNiell, M. (2008) Structuring time and questioning to achieve tactical awareness in games lessons, *Physical Education and Sport Pedagogy*, 13(3), pp. 231–250.

Metzler, M.W. (2005) *Instructional Models for Physical Education*. Scotdale, AZ: Holcomb Hathaway.

OfSTED (2004) *Subject Reports 2002/2003: Physical Education in Secondary School*. London: OfSTED.

—(2005) The annual report of Her Majesty's Chief Inspector of Schools 2004/05. Physical Education in Secondary Schools. www.OfSTED.gov.uk (accessed: 23 March 2009).

—(2008) *Curriculum Innovations in Schools. Age Group 5–19*. London: OfSTED.

O'Leary, N. (2008) Teaching Games for Understanding in learning to 'Outwit Opponents', *Physical Education Matters*, 3(4), pp. 18–20.

Papaioannou, A. and Goudas, M. (1999) Motivational climate of the physical education class (pp. 51–68). In Y. Vanden Auweele, F. Bakker, S. Biddle, M. Durand and R. Seiler (eds), *Psychology for Physical Educators*. Champaign, IL: Human Kinetics.

Parker, M. (1989) Academic learning time in physical education. In P. Darst, D. Zakrajsek, V. Mancini(eds), *Analyzing Physical Education and Sport Instruction*. Champaign, IL: Human Kinetics.

Pope, C. (2005) Once more with feeling: affect and playing with the TGfU model, *Physical Education and Sport Pedagogy*, 10(3), pp. 271–286.

Pye, J. (1988) *Invisible Children*. Oxford: Oxford University Press.

Qualifications and Curriculum Authority (2004) *High Quality Physical Education and Sport for Young People*. Nottinghamshire: DfES Publications.

Raab, M. (2007) Think SMART, not hard – a review of teaching decision making in sport from an ecological rationality perspective, *Physical Education and Sport Pedagogy*, 12(1), pp. 1–15.

Rink, J. (1996) Tactical and skill approaches to teaching sport and games [monograph], *Journal of Teaching in Physical Education*, 15(4).

SCAA (1995) *Planning the Curriculum at Key Stages 1 and 2*. London: School Curriculum and Assessment Authority.

Scanlan, T., Carpenter, P., Lobel, M. and Simons, J.P. (1993) Sources of enjoyment for youth sport athletes, *Pediatric Exercise Science*, 5(3), pp. 275–285.

Siedentop, D. and Tannehill, D. (2000) *Developing Teaching Skills in Physical Education*. Mountain View, CA: Mayfield.

Swann, J. (1999) Making better plans: problem-based versus objectives based planning (pp. 53–66). In J. Swann and J. Pratt (eds), *Improving Education: Realist Approaches to Method and Research*. London: Cassell.

—(2003) How science can contribute to the improvement of educational practice, *Oxford Review of Education*, 29(2), pp. 253–268.

Teaching and Learning Research Programme/Economic and Social Research Council (2007) Principles into practice: a teacher's guide to research evidence on teaching and learning. www.tlrp.org (accessed: 25 September 2008).

Theodoulides, A. (2003) Curriculum planning for inclusive physical education (pp. 15–32). In S. Hayes and G. Stidder (eds), *Equity and Inclusion in Physical Education and Sport*. London: Routledge.

Wankel, L.M. (1985) Personal and Situational factors affecting exercise involvement: the importance of enjoyment, *Research Quarterly for Exercise and Sport*, 56(3), pp. 275–282.

Weinberg, R.S. and Gould, D. (2002) *Foundations of Sport and Exercise Psychology*. Champaign, IL: Human Kinetics.

Williams, A. (1996) *Teaching Physical Education: Guide for Mentors and Students*. London: David Fulton.

Teaching Approaches

Andy Wild and Suzanne Everley

As new practitioners in a profession you will go through a process of establishing an approach to teaching that is reflective of your own pedagogic philosophy and the broader educational agenda within which you are operating. Developing such an approach may well involve challenging perceived wisdom in current practice in order to optimize learning for the young people with whom you are working. The extent to which the teacher is able to positively exploit the social, interactive possibilities of physical education is consistent with the degree of empowerment and ownership that individuals have towards their own progress. Here we will explore how established approaches to teaching some elements of physical education might be reviewed in light of the need to facilitate the development of independent, lifelong learners.

The teaching profession is one of constant critical self-reflection; as a practitioner you will continually take time, both formally and otherwise, to evaluate how effective you are within your teaching context and seek to improve your practice. As a good practitioner, within an environment of constant development, you will establish an approach to teaching that is reflective of your own pedagogic philosophy with respect to the social and environmental context in which you are working. Whilst you will inevitably be required to be responsive to a broader educational agenda, there will be certain essential elements to your approach to engaging with young people that will inform your action as a teacher. It is the process of establishing this approach – that is, 'who' you are as a teacher – that is of significance.

Much has been published in terms of the specifics of the processes through which young people are taught and their efficacy. Notions derived from the work of Mosston and Ashworth's spectrum of teaching styles (Mosston and Ashworth, 1986, 1990, 2002) have been widely explored and in themselves formed a central part of the debate as to how to most effectively engage learners. Further discussion centres on the motivation of young people and their interaction with the learning environment, both social and physical (Macfadyen and Bailey, 2002); all of which require attention when devising approaches to teaching. The ways in which the young person becomes motivated and is best disposed towards responding positively to the physical education context interacts with teaching styles; it is the optimization of these two factors that lead to the most effective learning and should inform your teaching approach.

Recent curricular developments have demanded that education be seen in the light of not only immediate effect, but sustained lifelong impact in terms of the willingness and ability to learn on a continued basis (CEC, 2001). Therefore, with respect to developing appropriate, effective and sustained approaches to teaching young people for lifelong learning, we are seeking to advocate a willingness to challenge existing practice.

This chapter focuses on an integrated child-centred teaching approach to (re)-engage learners in athletics (track and field) lessons. It traces the evolving practice that occurred in a secondary school following the appointment of a newly qualified physical education teacher.

The case study is matched by a review of selected relevant theory and discussion, which encourage the reader to consider – and question – their current practice; the text is complemented by Reflective Activities, which invite examination of the provision of athletics teaching within the school curriculum.

Reflections of a First Year Physical Education Teacher

. . .The crux of the problem was the practice I found in school after I'd qualified. The predominant teaching style used to deliver the athletics curriculum was a very formal command style. Pupils typically took their place in queues and waited their turn to run, jump or throw. It concerned me that some of the learners appeared so disillusioned; in fact a great many of them seemed to be being put off physical education by the experience. Surely that isn't right?

During my teacher training I'd been shown an alternative method for teaching athletics and I was keen to try it out. At first the other teaching staff were really sceptical and wary of my ideas; I was determined not to give up, so I sought permission to teach athletics differently *and to share my approach with colleagues. Thereafter the results were unbelievable – the class teaching became much more inclusive; many, many more children appeared to enjoy athletics lessons; the numbers attending athletics club after school increased; and the school team results didn't suffer.*

(First year secondary physical education teacher)

Reflection

Write a sentence that includes three adjectives, which highlight your qualities as a teacher and consider how they directly affect your *current teaching of track and field athletics activities.*

Would you agree that you currently include, engage and motivate *all* young people in your athletics lessons?

Developing Your Rationale

The efficacy of indirect teaching styles has been identified as being greatest in areas of activity that involve an element of creativity, that is, dance and gymnastics (Macfadyen and Bailey, 2006), but have been rather overlooked with respect to more formalized activities. For activities such as track and field athletics, discussion in literature strongly suggests that direct/command style teaching approaches (i.e. wherein the teacher is the sole/primary decision-maker), are necessary to achieved desired outcomes (Mawer, 1995 and Whitehead, 1997). Indeed the plethora of discourse regarding approaches to teaching games is a notably absent phenomenon with respect to athletics teaching. It is our contention that indirect approaches to teaching can be exploited in areas not traditionally considered creative (in this example, track and field athletics), and that it is also possible to actively combine direct and indirect approaches in the same lesson.

Arguably, there is a general movement within physical education teaching towards concept driven ideals; therefore approaches to teaching, which directly consider the learning environment as it exists in a social, interpersonal sense, take on a greater significance than they perhaps have previously. This, combined with a desire to create lifelong engagement with physical activity, underpins a philosophy that embraces approaches to teaching across the physical education curriculum to engage young people proactively in the process of their own learning.

Adult participation in physical activity is heavily dependent upon the social context in which it occurs (Laker, 2000); utilizing an approach in all areas of the physical education curriculum, which emphasizes peer interaction for teaching and learning provides a realistic anticipation of continued activity. Wragg (1996) and Laker (2000) seek to exemplify the importance of making lessons meaningful, however, experience is never without meaning and the potential of approaches to teaching to not only fail to positively engage young people, but to consequently alienate them from the learning process should not be overlooked. Therefore, although concepts of *enjoyment* as an appropriate goal of physical education form a moot point, the full engagement of the young person in the immediate learning process and continued engagement in physical activity is unlikely to be achieved without this. Consideration must be given to the ways in which the teacher's approach can make physical education positively meaningful *and* enjoyable for all young people.

Neil had always aspired to be a physical education teacher; during his school days he had always enjoyed physical education lessons and had regularly competed for his school in a number of sports. In his young twenties Neil fulfilled a lifetime ambition when he qualified as a secondary physical education teacher; his first post was in a large (11–18 years) school where he worked with five physical education colleagues, all of whom had been teaching for at least six years. The school has excellent physical education facilities and has a reputation locally, for fielding strong sporting teams – frequently winning local and regional competitions.

Neil has accepted that his all-round ability and enthusiasm for most sports and physical activity is not necessarily shared by everyone – something that had become apparent to him during his teacher training school-based experiences, where he met and taught young people who were not fully, nor positively engaged in physical education lessons. Although surprised by this, he was determined to learn more about the subject so he focused a final year assignment (in the form of an independent research project) to seek reasons why such attitudes presented; amongst the results of his small-scale investigation was a suggestion that when teachers use predominant didactic/command styles to deliver athletics, it can cause a barrier to the participation of non-sporty children. From that moment Neil embraced a personal philosophy based upon child-centred teaching and learning and he adopted a personal mantra that reminded him that 'Everything I ask a child to do should be worth doing'.

Reflection: Engaging Learners

Consider a recent lesson and answer these 5 questions:

1. When you planned the lesson did you consider the needs of all the learners?
2. Was the lesson appropriately resourced – staffing expertise and equipment/apparatus?
3. Can you identify any barriers that prevented you from engaging all learners?
4. Relevance and realism – did you include activities that were worth doing?
5. Who benefitted most from the lesson: You; all learners; groups of learners; individuals?

Barriers to Learning

In developing an approach to teaching we are engaged in making decisions regarding the 'powerful learning tools that both promote aspects of learning and prohibit others from occurring' (Whitehead, 1997, p. 131). Certain barriers need to be broken down in order to make the curriculum accessible to young people; it is the teachers' interpretation of what constitutes barriers and what constitutes facilitation that informs such decision-making. Barriers to participation – considered here to be those factors that prevent engagement with the learning environment itself – tend to revolve around concepts of the public and the hierarchical nature of the subject in terms of prioritizing ability, competition and power relations; that is, all concepts that can clearly be related to the phenomenon that is *sport*.

The relationship between didactic/command/direct styles of teaching similarly reinforce the hierarchical ordering that we see in sport. In particular, acknowledgement of success within track and field athletics taught in this way is necessarily measured by relative performance (highest, fastest, longest), rather than consideration of personal improvement or interactive process. Even where emphasis may be given by the teacher to the importance of personal progress, the public nature of both activity and its presentation expose a direct comparison to all others in the learning environment. In the extreme, long queues cause young people to perform one person at a time (e.g. high jump), frequently leading to a public exhibition of their limitations. This is exacerbated by the fact that some young people feel a sense of humiliation from performing in front of their peers in isolation and thus, may suffer further ridicule as a consequence of competing in this context. The elements of such an environment serve to mitigate against the engagement and motivation of some young people (arguably the majority). 'Simply put, children must feel good about themselves before they can learn effectively' (Laker, 2000, p. 94).

The concept of competition has often been considered pejorative in discussion about young people's participation in physical education; conversely, the absence of competition from the curriculum has stimulated a great deal of debate and consternation. However, what much discussion fails to adequately address is that competition is in itself an equivocal term. Competition 'can be against oneself, time or the environment' (Leah and Capel, 2000, p. 145) as well as another individual or group; concepts of co-operation and competition are not the mutually exclusive phenomena they are so readily perceived to be. What teaching approaches need to do in order to remove anxiety from competition, is to allow young people to create their own conditions for it to take place in; young people have a natural tendency to compete but the 'naturalness' of this is determined by the framework in which it exists. Therefore, allowing them to work in small groups, determine the members of that group and pace their engagement with the activity concerned, all serve to maximize the opportunity to take part in constructive competition.

This approach also facilitates the reduction in the influence of existing power hierarchies; those that are seen between teacher and learner and those that are seen between individuals and groups. If young people in school have the fundamental right of participation (Vickerman, 1997 and Talbot, 2007) then it is the teacher's obligation to make activities genuinely inclusive and accessible to all.

When Neil arrived at the school the athletics curriculum was based on a traditional track and field model. Lessons were discipline/event focused and the department policy was to record results (times and measurements) in every lesson, which the young people were expected to record in their Athletics Achievement Folder. The higher results were acknowledged by the staff and these were used to identify talent; moreover, the lesson-based achievements were used as a means of selecting school athletic teams. Neil was told that this way had always been successful because all the young people had a result for each particular event and the staff had a normative record, which enabled them to select strong school teams. In reality Neil observed that the significant majority of the young people did very little with the results. Most seemed not to care about personal bests and even fewer attended the school athletics club, which was perceived to be for the elite minority.

It was apparent that the year-on-year athletics curriculum lacked continuity and progression, and differentiation strategies didn't take account of knowledge, skills and understanding that had been acquired from previous athletics experiences; neither did the curriculum facilitate any personalized learning and nor did it support any opportunity for the young people to specialize in individual events or preferred disciplines. There was a significant reliance on command style delivery, whereby the teacher mostly told the whole class what to do, and the young people followed those instructions. In Neil's opinion, the school athletics curriculum was in fact putting young people off competing and participating, so he sought permission to employ an alternative teaching methodology that he'd been shown during his teacher training (shown below – Inclusive and Experiential Athletics). Thereafter, he used it with his classes in the 11–14 age group.

Inclusive and experiential athletics

Neil developed his practice upon the premise that young people had willingly participated within their peer group in all previous physical education lessons during the school year (for example, gymnastics, games and dance activities). They had been encouraged and expected to lead; evaluate; give feedback; and assess each other – hence Neil queried why the same/similar teaching styles weren't used to deliver athletics during the summer term?

Setting up teaching/learning contexts that mitigate the development of hierarchies – and thus empowering the majority – does create a complex set of variables regarding the evaluation and assessment of learning and performance. In any context, 'Pupils need to be made accountable and responsible for learning the task as set, and to work hard to achieve an appropriate level of learning' (Mawer, 1995, p. 104); this is particularly significant with a child-centred, peer assisted approach to teaching. Young people can be described as educational theorists who are actively interpreting and influencing the learning environment (Nicholls, 1992) and the utilization of such a teaching approach creates the potential to fully exploit this. Importance should be placed on the young person's current level of understanding and mastery (Mawer, 1995) and in best practice they are not compared directly to others. Young people can assess their environment and create thoughtfully constructed responses to this; linking learning between sessions and developing skills and understanding.

Young people have the critical acumen to evaluate their own experience (Groves and Laws, 2000) and their capacity for reflection enables the teacher to create a situation where everyone is engaging productively in an activity within the learning process. Where peer-assisted learning is used, the creation of a culture of accountability is significant for the individual and the group (Ward and Lee, 2005); in this way a young person is able to experience the relative success of the process in which they have been engaged and critically reflect on those elements of their interaction and participation that have lead to that success.

Reflection: Choice of Activities

Does your choice of activities (used within a lesson) build upon previous learning?
Are the activities sequential and relevant to every young person's stage of learning?
Do young people in your lessons understand the reason for the choice of activities?
Do learners have the opportunity to reflect upon their performances in each activity?

> Neil retained a central role to facilitate the learning; he planned a programme – which wasn't necessarily determined by weather conditions, school team competitions and/or teacher preferences/strengths – and included activities that placed the learners at the heart of the process, which enabled them to develop holistically. Responsibility and decision making was devolved to the participants by use of cue-cards/worksheets and/or teacher questions and prompts. For example, within one learning episode the participants engage in three different complimentary tasks/activities (i.e. run, jump, throw). The groups can be formed according to different and appropriately considered determinates: experience, ability, previous knowledge etc.; and the teacher prepares a safe working environment, in which the young people explore concepts, resolve problems and work to refine their performance and understanding by using evaluation and improvement strategies – using the same processes in fact, that they have employed in other/previous activity areas of the physical education curriculum.

It would be necessary, of course, for the teacher to set and affirm the standards that are expected in respect of behaviour, attitudes to learning, working with others etc.; however, given that athletics is mostly taught in the summer term as an outside activity, it is likely that the young people have already become accustomed to the teachers rules, routines and expectations in physical education lessons. Importantly, where safety issues arise due to the handling of specific and specialized athletic equipment, the teacher will complete an appropriate risk assessment and s/he should make the necessary adjustments; for example, one group may have teacher-led supervision regarding the safe use of a javelin, but could resolve responses to specific throwing techniques from stimulus other than directed teacher orders (e.g. cue-cards with sub-themes that give young people 'things to do', 'things to try' and 'things to talk about'). In this example, where the perceived and identified risk is higher, the teacher will be present to ensure safe handling, including throwing and retrieval of the implement. Meanwhile a separate group(s) can use similar cue-cards to meet outcomes in other disciplines; for example, to establish an individual run up for use in long jump or triple jump or timing reaction speed during reciprocated sprint start progressions. The positioning of the teacher enables a wide field of vision to be taken over the whole class – in the same way s/he would ensure peripheral vision to enable intervention over a class taking part in medium/high risk activities such as scrum progressions in rugby or flight themes in gymnastics.

The smaller group sizes facilitate increased participation, focused feedback (from teacher and peers) and thus, quicker individual improvement/progression – than might happen if the whole lesson was given over to throwing, where the teacher takes a position to control the safe sending and collection of a javelin by a large number of young people who appear to wait their turn in a queue to *have their go* (a practice that is not uncommon on many school sports fields).

Empowering Learners

It is significant that the potential for learning embraces the technical skills and capabilities associated with the activity and that it extends beyond this to socio-affective development; simultaneously giving rise to the potential to establish an enjoyable learning environment for the young people. Creating formalized learning environment, so often associated with the teaching of track and field athletics, removes the activity from the sense of play that makes activities so enjoyable for young people (and adults). The essence of play should not be lost 'when the formal social interaction of children becomes the formal delivery of education' Laker (2000, p. 29). The potential for enjoyment makes young people much more likely to take part in activities and extend their participation beyond school (Carroll and Loumidis, 2001 and Piotrowski, 2000). The most effective teaching actively engages young people in all stages of the learning process.

Leah and Capel (1997) identify that the social context in which young people are taught significantly affects their learning and Laker (2000) identifies that social outcomes are considered important in their assessment of the efficacy of a lesson; young people have a pre-existing social agenda and actively seek social interaction. Therefore, developing a teaching approach that allows for purposeful engagement with others is likely to have greater impact on learning.

Reflection: Delivery

Does your style of delivery allow all learners to engage in the activity to their full potential?
Does the style of delivery enable all the learners to progress?
Does the style of delivery empower the young people to share in their learning?
How do you deal with learner differences?

Contemporary approaches to games teaching (Sport Education and Teaching Games for Understanding) are child-centred: the teacher sets learning outcomes; the young people work collaboratively to solve problems; and they are actively engaged in their learning. The characteristics of these approaches can be successfully extended to other physical education activities.

Young people have a working consciousness that determines their focus whilst taking part in physical education and where they feel socially confident and physically competent (or at least, unthreatened) they are most able to concentrate on tasks set. Attitudes towards learning particular activities shape emotional responses to the environment. The extent to which individuals can affiliate with the learning context in which they are placed is important; moreover, when that is complemented by a sense of enjoyment, the affiliation is heightened.

If the teacher aims to create self-motivated individuals – who are likely to maintain involvement in physical activity beyond the school, in terms of both further participation outside of the classroom whilst of school age and subsequent continued participation as an adult – then child-centred learning needs to be considered as both a process and an objective. Child-centred learning should therefore be an aim of the curriculum itself, that is, the young person conceptualizes the notion of learning as a valuable experience and internalizes the processes through which they can achieve this.

Neil adopted a small-group/child-centred approach and immediately felt that the young people in his classes were purposely engaged and included in the Athletics lessons. He elicited further evidence by questioning the young people and found that they thought they had progressed because they had enjoyed the lessons and liked working with and supporting their friends. They also enjoyed the autonomous challenges presented on the cue-cards.

Neil shared his findings with colleagues at a department staff meeting and used a demonstration lesson to exemplify his teaching/delivery style. The teachers were invited to compare and question their current delivery and it was agreed that long queues of young people, waiting their turn to run, jump or throw, was something to avoid in physical education lessons (although it was found that that was in fact the dominant past and current practice). Thereafter the initial doubts and concerns gave way to an agreement to use the alternative teaching approach and during the latter part of the summer term Neil collaborated with his colleagues to assist their planning and delivery of Athletics lessons. The academic year concluded with a formal review of the physical education curriculum; the overwhelming consensus was that the athletics curriculum delivery had been far more inclusive (and enjoyable) for the pupils – and staff – and that progression and learning was more evident. Furthermore, the school representative Athletics teams had still acquitted themselves well at local competitions and the numbers of young people voluntarily attending the after-school athletics club had grown appreciably. The scenario, it was agreed, was a win-win situation and the department agreed to support Neil to plan a full and comprehensive programme to implement in future years.

Reflection: Next Steps

Review the current provision of track and field athletics in your school; you might start by sharing this chapter with colleagues that you work with and eliciting a response from them.

A staff and pupil survey may help to inform your future action; you may wish to find dedicated meeting time to discuss your findings and plan ahead.

Consider these questions and record your progress:

1. Where are we now? (Current situation)
2. What are we intending to change? (Future targets)
3. How are we going to get there? (Strategies)
4. What will we need to get there? (Resources)
5. What milestones will we have to meet? (Timescale)
6. What will we see to show that we've made a difference? (Evidence)

Concluding Comments

Within a child-centred approach to teaching, the teacher's role may appear to be minimized. Whilst this is arguably the case when considering the volume of teacher input, in practice, the role of the teacher becomes much more critical; s/he may appear to be teaching less, however well timed intervention is appropriately given to support pupil learning, which is far more effective than extended teacher input where the young person has less opportunity to process their thoughts.

Establishing child-centred, explorative teaching approaches in areas of the physical education curriculum that have a history and tradition of being taught in direct/command styles (such as track and field athletics) is a radical shift in philosophy and practice. The management of change (of process) is likely to present challenges and may even cause tension amongst colleagues. It is the contention of the authors however, that change in many instances is both desirable and necessary. The following key links (see 'Learning More', below) and the concluding reflection activity may prove helpful in informing and guiding your next steps.

Learning More

The Qualification and Curriculum Authority in England has conducted a physical education and school sport (PESS) investigation, which has shown that improving the quality of PESS can have a remarkable impact on young people and their schools. The schools involved in the PESS investigation aimed to ensure that all of their pupils spend a minimum of two hours each week on high quality physical education and school sport (PESS). At the same time, each school selected one or more whole-school improvement objectives that it would like to achieve through investing in PESS (ranging from improved progress and attainment in PESS, to improved behaviour and attendance). For further information visit www.qca.org.uk/pess.

Elevating Athletics is a set of resources designed to place running, jumping and throwing at the heart of school physical education and to support teachers in delivering athletic activity in an inclusive, exciting and engaging manner. Elevating Athletics is written by physical education experts with extensive experience of teaching and coaching athletics at school, club and international level. Elevating Athletics is written to conform to curriculum requirements in England, Northern Ireland, Scotland and Wales. It has been delivered to every State school in the UK. For further information visit www.ukathletics.net.

Hayes et al. (2000) provides self-assessment strategies and ideas that encourage teachers to reflect actively on their own professional practice and to enrich their day-to-day work. Topics covered include short- and long-term planning, using resources, communication, questioning techniques, motivating young people, assessment and evaluation.

References

Carroll, B. and Loumidis, J. (2001) Children's perceived competence and enjoyment in physical education and physical activity outside school, *European Physical Education Review*, 7(1), pp. 24–43.

Commission of the European Communities (CEC) (2001) *Communication from the Commissions: Making a European Are of Lifelong Learning a Reality*. Brussels: European Commission.

Groves, S. and Laws, C. (2000) Children's experiences of physical education, *European Journal of Physical Education*, 5(1), pp. 19–27.

Hayes, L. Nikolic, V. and Cabaj, H. (2000) *Am I teaching well? Self-evaluation strategies for effective teachers*. Exeter: Learning Matters.

Laker, A. (2000) *Beyond the Boundaries of Physical Education*. London: Routledge.

Leah, J. and Capel, S. (2000) Competition and co-operation in physical education (pp. 144–158). In S. Capel and S. Piotrowski (eds), *Issues in Physical Education*. London: Routledge Falmer.

Macfadyen, T. and Bailey, R. (2002) *Teaching Physical Education 11–18*. London. Continuum.

Mawer, M. (1995) *The Effective Teaching of Physical Education*. London: Longman.

Mosston, M. and Ashworth, S. (1986) *The Effective Teaching of Physical Education*. London, Merrill.

—(1994) *Teaching Physical Education*. Third edition. Oxford: Maxwell Macmillan.

—(2002) *Teaching Physical Education*. Fifth edition. London: Benjamin Cummings.

Nicholls, J.G. (1992) Students as educational theorists (pp. 267–286). In D. Schunk and J. Meece (eds), *Students Perceptions in the Classroom*. Hillsdale, NJ: Erlbaum.

Piotrowski, S. (2000) Health and life-long physical activity (pp. 170–187). In S. Capel and S. Piotrowski (eds), *Issues in Physical Education*. London: Routledge Falmer.

Talbot, M. (2007) Policy matters: quality, *Physical Education Matters*, 2(2), p. 6.

Vickerman, P. (1997) Knowing your pupils and planning for different needs (pp. 139–157). In S. Capel and S. Piotrowski (eds), *Issues in Physical Education*. London: Routledge Falmer.

Ward, P. and Lee, M. (2005) Peer assisted learning in physical education: a review of theory and research, *Journal of Teaching Physical Education*, 24, pp. 205–225.

Whitehead, M. (1997) Teaching styles and teaching strategies (pp. 130–138). In S. Cape (ed.), *Learning to Teach Physical Education in the Secondary School*. London: Routledge.

Wragg, E. (ed.) (1996) *Classroom Teaching Skills*. London: Routledge.

8 Assessment for Learning

Andrew Frapwell

Research by Black and Wiliam at the turn of the twentieth century developed a wide acceptance that there was an unequal power sharing in traditional learning and teaching relationships. What has developed is the notion that the responsibility for learning should be shared by the teacher and learner wherever possible. This shift views good teaching, as being centred on the facilitation of student learning. The focus of attention is firmly upon the student, and teacher activity is of value or of interest only in respect of what it enables students to achieve. The shift to a focus on the learner initially brought about a plethora of types of assessment that happen *after* learning has taken place. This manifested itself with a teacher obsession to transform every bit of progress a student makes into marks, symbols or grades. This over emphasis on Assessment *of* Learning has now shifted to an emphasis on Assessment *for* Learning (AfL). Effective assessment is viewed as assessment information that is used to inform and direct teacher and student efforts in learning and learning improvement. In particular research carried out by Black and Wiliam (1999) found that students taught by teachers who used this 'assessment for learning' approach would achieve in six or seven months what would otherwise take a year.

The Name Game – Introducing Assessment

When my eldest son first started school at 4 years of age, he participated in a number of different project activities that helped his learning for reading and writing. He made shapes of his name, he used different colours to shade each letter and he glued these onto paper and project folders. In dance and gymnastics he 'wrote' his name on the floor by following appropriate pathways and using different methods – running, skipping, jumping, hopping, crawling or rolling. Outside, the school playground had various painted letter pathways marked for children to follow and in the Forest School (an outdoor classroom) he was able to create his name using mud, sticks, grass and stones. He 'researched' the meaning and history of his name using the internet and he was required to ask his parents why he was given his particular name, recounting 'his story' to others in class circle time. Parents were seen very much as partners in the learning process and much conversation was generated by optional home learning tasks.

One of the books that I remember him reading aloud to us at home – speaking the individual letters phonetically and on occasion acting out the objects or actions associated with the alphabet – was called *Matthew A. B. C*, written by Peter Catalanotto (2005). Mrs Tuttle, a teacher, has 25 children in her class. They are all named Matthew. The school principal wonders how Mrs Tuttle tells them apart. She finds it quite simple. Starting with the letter 'A', each Matthew has something special about him. For example, Matthew A is extremely affectionate, Matthew B loves Band-Aids and Matthew C has cowlicks. This continues letter by letter, through the alphabet until Matthew Y who can yodel. One day the principal brings another boy to join the class – bet you can't guess his name!

All of the planned activities and opportunities outlined helped my son and his class friends to process information in several ways to learn to read and write. Social connections with others and emotional connections to their learning were promoted. The experiences also provided rich, stimulating, supportive and diverse environments. Perhaps as important, the learning provision planned was relevant or personal to the individual, it was meaningful and it was coherent. Catalanotto's (2005) children's book also serves to illustrate that each individual is unique. Learning is diverse and different for each learner and it is exactly this diversity that provides innumerable opportunities for expanding learning and making it coherent and interesting. In every sense the learning examples shared here are provided for learning to be maximized and clearly position the learner at the heart of the process. At this stage of learning the standard assessment method was required to be 80 per cent through observing children play. Any gaps in learning that teachers became aware of were subsequently targeted and provided for. Assessment was an integral part of a genuine process *for* learning. There were no tests. Learning was rich fun and enjoyable.

> **Reflection**
>
> - How do you currently perceive assessment and is this reflected in how you use it?
> - What do you understand by the phrase 'teaching to the test' or teaching to the grade or level descriptor?
> - What are the benefits or limitations of approaching the teaching of physical education in this way?
> - What is AfL?

Assessment – What's in a Name?

Just as the name 'Matthew' conjured up various associations with personality or behaviours of an individual for Mrs Tuttle, so the term 'Assessment' conjures up different meanings according to national, regional, local and individual contexts and philosophies, the theoretical frameworks of the practitioners and researchers and understanding of the process of learning. These are all critical in determining our perception and understanding of assessment.

In regularly facilitating teacher learning in assessment workshops in the United Kingdom and through observed practice whilst visiting schools in the USA and Europe, the responses noted from teachers to the question; 'What is Assessment?' tends to fall into three broad categories: Monitoring, recording and reporting learner achievement; testing; and allocating learners a level of attainment or a grade. On reflection the first of these isn't assessment – these are activities that happen *after* assessment has taken place. The second, testing, is but *one method* of assessment; and allocating a grade is predominantly carried out because it is *required at the end of a process*. Further probing questioning demonstrates that teachers really do struggle to explain what the level or grade actually means and this is further compounded when asked to explain the term physical education and teaching as distinct from sport and sports coaching. What are usually described are isolated activities that are engaged with and that a teacher teaches a range of sports, whereas a coach tends to specialize in one sport. This rather limited response suggests that as a profession we remain unsure of the knowledge that distinguishes us as teachers and teachers' knowledge in physical education can be just as perplexing (Cassidy and Rossi, 1999). 'What's in a name?' therefore is of utmost importance if we are to understand the assessment process or indeed what we are actually assessing. Using my son's experience, he was learning *in* and *through* physical education. He was learning to travel using a variety of methods *in* physical education, but also learning to recognize and shape letters *through* physical education. This adds another dimension to learning and the opportunities that might be provided need to be coherently planned in the context of a child's whole education. Physical education cannot be viewed as isolated. Whilst the remainder of the chapter builds information and understanding in and around AfL in physical education, it is beyond the remit and boundaries of this chapter brief to explore exactly what constitutes physical education.

Reflection

When planning, how do you/might you ensure that:

- Learning is focused on whole curriculum aims/approaches?
- Learning is coherent for students across the curriculum subjects?
- Learning is planned in and through physical education?

How does your physical education programme inspire and challenge all of your learners?

How do you gather information to check that student learning is strategic, coherent, meets any statutory requirement and meets student's needs?

How do you use assessment to inform your planning?

How do you use assessment to inform your future learning and teaching?

The Burden of a Name

The term 'assessment' stems from the Latin word 'Assessare' which means 'to sit beside'. This meaning originally appeared in the Encyclopedia Britanicca in 1911 (Encyclopedia Brittanica website 2009). It was a Roman term applied to a trained lawyer who 'sat beside' a governor of a province or other magistrate to guide or instruct him in the administration of the Laws. The Lawyer was never the judge, yet this is the meaning the word 'Assessment' has taken on, largely due to the way it was misunderstood by its early promoters and how it has been politicised by many of the world's governments.

The Burden of Proof – Assessment as Proving

There is an inevitable danger that tests, which originally might have been designed to assess learner *progress,* have become the foundations of curricula. In physical education, this has manifested itself in a whole battery of 'sports' tests, fitness tests or skill tests. One example in England is a Multi-skills programme designed to augment the basic curriculum in out of school hours learning and develop children's physical skills. Unfortunately it is often taught as curriculum physical education, and performance on the skills test at the end is used to contribute to a grade or level. This limiting approach can result in very narrow uninspiring curricula. The misguided need to 'prove' that assessment is taking place has also unfortunately led to excessive test practice and more frequent testing. As every farmer knows, continuously weighing one's produce does not hasten its readiness for market. Tests and testing have become synonymous with proof and proving. This 'high stakes' testing is not always a bad thing as in the absence of testing children sometimes have a lower opinion of themselves, but it can also cause considerable anxiety in teachers and learners (Green, 2006). This anxiety is especially prevalent in student teachers and new teachers when assessing movement and physical skills. In addressing this concern there is a danger that these skills are over-taught and over-assessed (and this is different to providing opportunity to practice and learn) which is exactly the wrong thing to do. The result can be a narrow sports outcomes approach to the subject of physical education. This issue is compounded by the fact that movement and physical skills are transitory at various stages of a young person's development and the danger is that too frequent assessment results in the generation of too much information that demonstrates regression as well as progression. This can further knock the confidence of practitioners. The power of the improving feature of assessment, the sitting beside and guiding aspect has, and is still being neglected – or perhaps more poignantly – is not being recognized, understood and implemented.

Throughout the past 20–30 years efforts have been made to modify assessment to better convey meanings and purposes. The profession distinguished between formative, diagnostic, summative and evaluative assessment to try to clarify when and why assessment is carried out (Task Group on Assessment and Testing, 1987). Assessment cycles were developed in order to imply that assessment was a continuous process rather than a discrete event. Initial words were added to clarify the purpose when referring to teacher assessment or learner assessment. The notion of authentic assessment evolved in an attempt to make assessment tasks or tests more real, more meaningful and more relevant; and these tasks also helped provide a range of assessment evidence as 'proof' of any grades allocated. The phrase 'Assessment for Learning' grew from a move to 'rebrand' assessment in order to delineate its true purpose. The noun, however, and hence the central focus, is always assessment. This word continues to convey misleading meanings and images in spite of modifying words or phrases. There is no mention in the literature that one of the purposes of assessment was accountability, although there are plenty of references implying that assessment informs the process of being held accountable as a profession. And so the lines are drawn and assessment has continued to struggle – against these early misunderstandings – to gain both respectability and worth.

Shifting the Burden – Assessment as Improving

In the past 20 years there has been a progressive move from a focus on the teacher to a focus on the learner. This is drawn from the work of Lusted (1986), who focused on the processes through which knowledge is produced such as thought, discussion, writing, debate and exchange. He believed that how one teaches, although of central interest, is inseparable from what is being taught and how one learns. This view of education that has come to dominate mainstream educational thinking, particularly during the 1990s and 2000s, asserts that all knowledge is constructed as a result of cognitive processes within the human mind (Klenowski, 1996). This thinking built on the constructivist work of Bruner (1960) who proposed four main themes. These themes were based around how structure, learner readiness, intuitive and analytical thinking, and motives for learning should be made central to teaching and learning. Bruner (1960) argued that the teaching and learning of structure is more than simple mastery of facts and techniques and it is this learning that helps individuals make sense of later revisited learning. The learning of structure is important to the notion of learner readiness in that 'difficult learning' can be taught effectively to children at any stage of development in some form. It is these high teacher expectations of learner readiness and the learning of structure that promote opportunity for learners to make intuitive leaps without going through the formal analytical progressive steps which can often slow progress and independent thought. If teachers seek to promote this type of engagement with the curriculum content and children are excited to learn because the material is presented in an 'irresistible' way then this provides a better motive for learning than external grades, numbers or levels. From this conceptual framework Bruner (1960) formulated his *spiral curriculum* where concepts, knowledge, skills and understanding are constantly revisited in a process model of learning.

What has developed is the notion that the responsibility for learning should be shared by the teacher and learner wherever possible. This shift views good planning and teaching, as being centred on the facilitation of student learning. The focus of attention is firmly upon the learner, and teacher activity is of value or of interest only in respect of what it enables learners to achieve. This is occurring globally, and across all subjects as the nature of teaching and learning is changing.

In physical education for learning terms this has meant a shift from 'planning content' and 'teaching for coverage' and the continued assessment of this, to a new look at the relationship between how we select and order experiences for young people around their needs; how they think and process information about learning in physical education in order to improve their performances; and how AfL practices can become embedded in these processes. A lack of

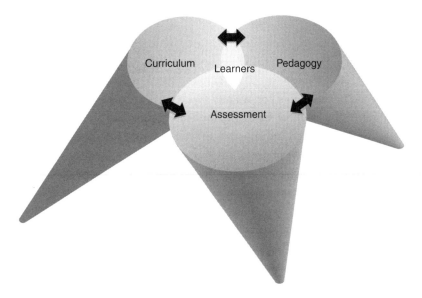

Figure 8.1 The curriculum-assessment-pedagogy inter-relationship (adapted from Black, 2006).

knowledge and understanding about this relationship can therefore narrow and inhibit planning, which in turn can narrow and inhibit the way we teach, and both can impact adversely on assessment opportunity. The importance of the inter-relationship therefore, between three key education components: Curriculum, Assessment and Pedagogy, cannot be ignored.

Key to this inter-relationship is that learners are at the heart of everything we do. Figure 8.1 promotes a torchlight analogy. If planned separately the three components can appear isolated and unrelated to learners who are in the dark. The more effective our practice and focus on learner's and learning, and the more we understand and can harness the creative tension between the three components, the more concentric the circles will be,

---

Reflection

- How do you currently use knowledge of your learners to plan curriculum, assessment or pedagogical experiences?
- How have your curriculum, assessment and pedagogical practice evolved over the course of your professional career?
- How critical has your assessment practice been in advancing teaching and learning and improving curriculum for *all* learners?

---

the brighter the focus, the more enjoyable the experiences for learners, the greater the achievement:

- Curriculum – what we select for the pupils to learn – designed and planned around their needs.
- Pedagogy – the ways in which curriculum is delivered based on learner needs.
- Assessment – used to advance teaching and learning and improve curriculum, as well as 'judging' how well pupils have progressed because of our curriculum provision and pedagogical practices.

Easing the Burden: Beyond the Pale

Ultimately it should be the school community that co-constructs the educational experience with students. While the essential standards for achievement and attainment around which the curriculum is constructed are mostly government specified, the need for flexibility and personalization need to be understood. It is these elements that can help schools and individual teachers to provide deep, rich and engaging learning experiences and opportunities for all young people. Success in learning is more likely if the curriculum that is planned and the way it is taught excites and challenges young people. A clearer focus on AfL will increase learners' engagement, and enable them to show what they can do opening doors to higher achievement (QCA, 2008). This is an obvious shift away from curricula and pedagogy that is driven by assessment and clearly places the learner at the heart of the process. In England a significant shift in supporting this process has been the removal of standardized assessment tests at age 14.

The removal of testing can help promote greater freedom and personalization and reduce the grading function of assessment, but these are not necessarily prerequisites to promoting the learning function of assessment. In promoting the learning function of assessment education is attempting to move beyond the 'pale' uninspiring curricula that often result from teaching to the test, to deep enriching learning experiences and opportunities for learners.

Developing strategy

The strategy for any school, physical education department/faculty or teacher ought to be to make AfL more widespread, systematic and consistent. This means:

- effective systems and processes in place that actually lead to informing learning and teaching in some way and that promote the decoupling of assessment from accountability;
- teachers who know and understand the concepts, principles and processes involved with progression *in* and *through physical education*;
- learners who know where they are in their learning, who work towards ambitious targets, who know how to get there and who know how they are progressing and;
- parents and carers who are involved with this process in order to support children.

When pupils and their teachers have a really good understanding of where they are in their learning, where they need to go next and how best to get there – which is what AfL is all about – then a real difference is evident in learners (Assessment Reform Group, 1999). This process is important because it promotes: ownership and engagement of learning; learners (not just young people) who are more self-aware; learners who are confident to innovate or make intuitive leaps; and above all parallel and mutually supportive *for* learning processes. These features highlight assessment as an integral part of the (spiral) curriculum (Bruner, 1960).

Implications for practice

The shift to a focus on the learner initially brought about a plethora of types of assessment that happen *after* learning has taken place. Information or evidence if gathered and recorded by the teacher is usually transformed into marks or grades. Performance with others is often compared and it is reviewed in the context of past learning. This over-emphasis on 'Assessment *of* Learning' has now shifted to an emphasis on 'Assessment *for* Learning'.

A useful starting point to embedding assessment processes into everyday practice is to focus on the quality of communication with the learner. The more effective communication is with the learner and the more effective teachers are at developing learner communication with their peers, then the better student learning and progress will be. This starts with understanding of the importance of the smallest interaction between teacher and learner and the involvement of all learners in this process. This '*Day to day*' *communication* is important for providing information that can be used in making decisions about immediate next steps in children's learning and this can be drawn from a wide range of specific contexts as well as focusing on subject content matter. Limited interaction with learners could focus solely on knowledge and facts of performing an accurate throwing action for example, but this ignores knowledge of structural learning, irresistible and authentic learning and also knowledge of the learner in terms of personal development, emotional needs, learning and thinking skills and preferred learning styles.

It is the quality of this smallest interaction, pupil involvement in peer- and self-assessment and the target setting and review process beyond numbers or grades, that can all help raise learner aspirations, learner progress and ultimately the attainment of higher standards (QCA, 2008). When combined with the challenging yet sensitive and supportive sharing of assessment information it can lead to greater *learner confidence* and *learner commitment*. Four types of interactions, derived from research into effective teacher practice were suggested as being central, though not exclusive in promoting or accelerating learning at the 'day to day level' (Black and Wiliam, 1998). These should not be viewed as standalone, rather inter-related elements:

- questioning and dialogue;
- feedback;
- sharing criteria;
- peer assessment.

Eliciting information through questioning and dialogue

Common practice by teachers often centres on question and answer (Q and A) techniques. There is a danger with this method that young learners simply guess the answer they think the teacher wants. This is associated strongly with a planning approach to physical education that focuses on content and coverage of skill rather than what is appropriate for the stage of the learner related to a broad range of physical education outcomes. In other words, the more limited the curriculum experience, the more limited the curriculum. In these instances learners respond to a large majority of teacher-posed *factual questions* (Frapwell and Jarrett, 2003), which usually involve learners repeating information to the teacher that they were given earlier in the lesson – 'you hold the racket with a v-grip Miss.' Questioning that promotes dialogue between learners (Q and D) – or *process questions* – provides opportunity for learners to process information related to the experience they have just had. A question that probes the effectiveness of different types of defence in a games activity, for example, requires learners to reflect on their experiences and use evidence to inform future practice. Improvement might be targeted at individual skill, communication or types of defence (zone/person to person) and decisions will be different appropriate to the opposition or appropriate to participant's level of fitness. Where this type of questioning was used predominantly, teachers not only gained insight into learner's thoughts and ideas – which helped them plan future tasks for learners – but they also observed significant improvement in performances. Further benefits included improvement in learner attitudes, confidence and commitment to learning as a result of the opportunities provided (Frapwell, 2005). Developing *questioning skills* that engage learners cognitively and encourage them to reflect on their own and others work and make decisions about where they progress next are vital to learner and teacher understanding and progress.

Providing feedback with emphasis on how to improve

In order to progress and succeed, children need appropriate and supportive feedback on their learning. This can be received in a number of various forms or channels – visual (written, image, non-verbal), auditory or kinaesthetic. Feedback isn't always from teacher to learner but can be provided through peer- and self-assessment methods. The more effective the feedback the better the progress made. Feedback is something that (physical education) teachers are surrounded by and involved in every day, yet it is poorly analysed and poorly used (Askew and Lodge, 2000).

Consider the following feedback (adapted from Gipps et al., 2000):

- Rewards and sanctions for good/poor behaviour;
- Rewards and sanctions for effort/lack of effort;
- Personal expressions of approval/disapproval.

The above examples are as a result of making decisions about learner responses to tasks or instructions given.

Consider these:

- Telling children they are right or wrong;
- Describing why a performance is correct or incorrect;
- Describing why an answer is right or wrong;
- Telling children what they have achieved or have not achieved.

The above are examples of using knowledge produced from 'making assessments of observed performance' to feedback in a declarative or descriptive way to learners. Declarative knowledge addresses the gap between 'effect' and 'ideal effect'. Assessment criteria are starting to become visible, but the description is still only of the end result. Feedback on *'knowing that'* is typified at this level by the 'run faster' 'balance longer' or 'concentrate harder' comment. The step progress here, however, is that practice has moved from a stage where subjective decisions about learner responses are made, to a point where descriptions of pupil decisions or performances are provided. This level of feedback is still rather limited in terms of impacting on learner progress as it doesn't specify *'how to'* improve.

Consider the next level:

- Specifying or implying a better way of doing something;
- Setting targets for improvement and sharing criteria;

- Negotiating targets and ways of achieving them;
- Questioning pupils to task them to suggest targets and implement strategies.

The previous examples offer knowledge about '*how to*' or the use of procedural knowledge, which shares exactly what you have to do to achieve targets. Learners are made partners in the learning process. Criteria are transparent, challenge is provided and expectations are continuously being revised. Going further and providing the 'why?' before the 'how?' addresses the gap between cause and effect and learners will benefit enormously if teachers paid more attention to information and processes provided to close this gap. When applied to a ground stroke in tennis, for example, many beginners often mis-time the shot closing the racquet face – the cause – resulting in the ball to misdirect – the effect. Understanding the 'why?' promotes structural learning and thinking about why something happened which promotes engagement in a process of considering how it might be corrected – such as techniques to keep the racquet face open and perpendicular to the flight of the ball.

Helping learners understand quality criteria

The obvious prerequisite is that teachers understand quality criteria before they can share it effectively with learners (see also feedback). This again raises the issue of teacher knowledge and understanding of what it is to be physically educated. The following '*If – Then*' sequencing describes what is termed assessment alignment and is adapted from ideas in my own early career.

IF   There are *clearly defined* long-, medium- and short-term learning objectives and outcomes . . .

THEN   There are clearly defined long, medium and short-term *assessment criteria* for assessing pupils' *achievement and attainment* which can be used to make decisions about future learning and teaching.

IF   There are *clear progressions* in the learning objectives and outcomes outlined in a scheme or curriculum plan, and these are reflected in the content of their associated units and lessons . . .

THEN   There are assessment criteria for assessing learners' *progress* as part of the learning and teaching process.

IF   Learners are provided with opportunities to *demonstrate their learning in authentic Physical Education contexts* . . .

THEN   Teachers will have *evidence* on which to make assessment decisions and judgements about pupils in physical education.

IF   Learning objectives and outcomes are progressive and *describe stages of learning* from an anticipated base level to learning commensurate with expected levels for a particular stage (not age) . . .

THEN   There are assessment criteria which can be applied to and used to *describe the range of achievement and attainment* from the less able to the most able learners.

IF   These processes are *embedded* and *effectively employed* in school or departments/faculty systems, processes and practice . . .

THEN   We have *sufficient data and evidence to gauge the impact* of any improved teacher practice (re pedagogy and curriculum planning) on pupil progression, achievement or attainment related to department/faculty, school, state or government priorities, as well as information about the effectiveness of teacher professional development.

Peer- and self-assessment

Improvement in learning can really start to develop when all learners in the class are 'teachers'. Self- or peer-assessment requires the learner to identify gaps and to give feedback on their own or others work. Making this type of judgement involves having an understanding of the criteria and a concept of quality, and it also involves practice. The learner must therefore have the knowledge and the ability to respond to feedback and make changes to work. The intermediary step is negotiated or collaborative assessment with the teacher – the teacher 'sits beside' the learner judge, and helps or instructs him – wasn't this the original meaning of the word? Essentially, learners will need to know and understanding what is required for a given task. This will also mean having the experience to make decisions about the quality of that work with reference to the criteria that the teacher specifies. The underpinning rationale of self- or peer-assessment is that it helps the learner to understand what s/he is doing (Sadler, 1989). It is a way of providing feedback which can be directly and immediately applied to the work in progress. When considered in this way, assessment becomes transparent as a focused form of communication with the learner. The more effective this communication with the learner, the better their progress will be. This illustrates the important inextricable link between pedagogy (teaching and learning) and assessment for learning.

Reflection

1. Map your current 'communication' practice to the following four key action continuums.
2. Discuss with colleagues the evidence from your practice you used in determining this 'point'.
3. Independently or collaboratively set targets as to 'what' you might develop.
4. Develop a rationale as to 'why' you should change.
5. Plan strategies as to 'how' you might develop.
6. As a result of any improved teacher outputs, what improved learner outcomes will you expect to see?

Four Progressive Key Actions:

1. Questioning

— — — — — — — — — — — — — — →

Question and answer
Is the question worth asking?

Question and dialogue
What is the learning purpose of the question?

⇨

2. Feedback

Feedback on behaviours	Descriptive	Analytical
Good, well done	*That was good because . . .*	*This is why and how you improve*

3. Feedback Understanding criteria

Sports outcomes	Criteria shared clearly	Aligned physical education outcomes

4. Feedback Peer and self-assessment

Teacher directed	Collaborative	Independent
Controlled – observe and imitate		*Reflective – analyse and innovate*

Concluding Remarks

Re-emphasizing the learning function of Assessment and de-emphasizing the grading function are necessities if the process of Assessment, integral to curriculum and pedagogical processes, is to be hailed a key driver in raising standards in physical education and assume it's true identity. Central to this shift is teacher knowledge and understanding of physical education in the wider context of learning for life, and the vital role they should play in the whole process – one of the 'sitting beside' the learner and guiding or instructing them. It is the effectiveness of this 'day to day' communication with the learner that helps learners make immediate progress, and develops them as learners who are an integral part of the whole process.

AfL involves creating an ethos in a physical education authentic context where talk and dialogue about learning are central to the day-to-day communication. Assessment can be a very powerful tool in supporting, motivating, enthusing and engaging *teachers and learners* in their commitment to learning in physical education. To that end, professional development to equip new and existing teachers with the skills and vision to look beyond statutory requirements and personalize engaging experiences and opportunities in physical education for learning, with assessment and the learner at the heart of the process is required.

Learning More

There are some useful sources that map the topography of assessment promoting reader understanding (e.g. Lambert and Lines, 2000). Much of Black and Wiliam's research is very practicable and user-friendly from a teaching and learning perspective and the publication Black et al. (2003) really helps to contextualize the use and implementation of assessment used to accelerate learning *and* teaching practice and raise standards. When observed in this way the notion of parallel learning processes emerge, and Day and Sachs (2004) is a very useful source promoting teachers as learners first and explores effective CPD associating improved teacher outputs and improved outcomes for young people. Finally, Stoll et al. (2003) focus on learning, and expound the conditions for learning where AfL practice is essential for making learning 'visible' and promoting 'habits of mind'.

References

Askew, S. and Lodge, C. (2000) Gifts, ping-pong and loops – linking feedback and learning (pp. 1–18). In S. Askew (ed.) *Feedback for Learning*. London: Routledge.

Assessment Reform Group. (1999) *Assessment for Learning: Beyond the Black Box*. Cambridge: University of Cambridge School of Education, Assessment Reform Group.

Black, P. (2006) Assessment for and of Learning. Appendix 4 (pp. 30–34). In S. Tough and J. Reed (eds), *Curriculum, Assessment and Pedagogy: Beyond the 'standards agenda'*. London: Institute for Public Policy and Research.

Black, P. and Wiliam, D. (1998) *Inside the Black Box: Raising Standards through Classroom Assessment*. London: School of Education, King's College.

Black, P., Harrison, C., Lee, C., Marshall, B. and Wiliam, D. (2003). *Assessment for Learning: Putting It into Practice*. Maidenhead: Open University Press.

Bruner, J. (1960) *The Process of Education*. Cambridge, MA: Harvard University Press.

Cassidy, T. and Rossi, T. (1999) Knowledgeable teachers in physical education: a view of teachers' knowledge (pp. 188–202). In C. Hardy and M. Mawer (eds), *Learning and Teaching in Physical Education*. London: Falmer Press.

Catalanotto, P. (2005) *Matthew ABC*. New York: Athenian Books.

Day, C. and Sachs, J. (2004). *International Handbook on the Continuing Professional Development of Teachers*. Maidenhead: Open University Press.

Frapwell, A. (2005) From practice to principles (pp. 55–62). In C. Casbon and L. Spackman (eds), *Assessment for Learning in Physical Education*. Leeds: Coachwise.

Frapwell, A. and Jarrett, H. (2003) How can we use questioning to target understanding? Paper presented at the First Hawaii International Conference on Education. 7–10 January 2003. Hawaii.

Gipps, C., McCallum, B. and Hargreaves, E. (2000) *What Makes a Good Primary School Teacher? Expert Classroom Strategies*. London: Routledge Falmer.

Green, S. (2006) Curriculum, assessment and pedagogy (pp. 5–6). In S. Tough and J. Reed (eds), *Curriculum, Assessment and Pedagogy: Beyond the 'standards agenda'*. London: Institute for Public Policy and Research.

Lambert, D. and Lines, D. (2000). *Understanding Assessment: Purposes, Perceptions, Practice*. London: Routledge Falmer.

Leahy, S., Lyon, C., Thompson, M. and Wiliam, D. (2005) Classroom assessment: minute by minute, day by day, *Educational Leadership*, 63(3), pp. 19–24.

Lusted, D. (1986) Why pedagogy? *Screen*, 27(5), pp. 2–14.

Morreale, S.P. and Backlund, P.A. (1999) Assessment: coming of age, *Anatomy of Assessment*, Spring, pp. 22–23.

Qualifications and Curriculum Authority (QCA) (2008) http://curriculum.qca.org.uk/key-stages-3-and-4/developing-your-curriculum/new_opportunities/ (accessed: 16 March 2009).

Sadler, R. (1989) Formative assessment and the design of instructional systems, *Instructional Science*, 18(2), pp. 119–144.

Stoll, L., Fink, D., and Earl, L. (2003). *It's About Learning (and It's About Time): What's in It for Schools*. London: Routledge Falmer.

Task Group on Assessment and Testing (1987) National Curriculum: a report. London: DES.

9 Models of Pedagogy

Gary D. Kinchin

Research has demonstrated that instruction in physical education is commonly teacher-directed. To teach effectively for a broad range of learning outcomes teachers both need secure subject knowledge and the ability to use a wider range of instructional models. This chapter therefore provides an overview of some alternative models of curriculum and instruction which have been designed to place the learner actively and socially at the centre of the teaching and learning process. As we shall see each of the selected models have been found to lead to positive outcomes for pupils and have the potential to form a key part of a school physical education programme.

Introduction

Several teaching and learning models exist offering an alternative to what some have called the 'traditional' approach (Capel and Blair, 2007; Green, 2008). This traditional approach describes a teacher-directed form of instruction, based mostly around skill acquisition and performance in drills, operating across short units, within a multi-activity curriculum of a mostly games and sports orientation. Critiques of such programmes, specifically the degree to which they address inclusion and the physical activity needs of children and youth (in particular some girls and pupils of lower ability) have emerged (Ennis, 1996, 2000; Kirk, 2005). Despite major innovations in curriculum, including some at national level, some physical education teachers have not changed the way they teach (e.g. Green 1998, 2008; Curtner-Smith, 1999; Capel and Blair, 2007) and instead tend to reproduce a pedagogy that they themselves experienced as pupils. That a mostly teacher-directed 'picture' is felt to exist in many secondary schools (Byra, 2006) it is a curricular approach many readers may have experienced in their own schooling.

This is not to deny that command/teacher-directed forms of instruction do have their place within the curriculum and may be more appropriate where, for example, pupil safety is essential (e.g. the teaching of swimming or the introduction to archery) or learning early fundamental motor skills. This chapter is concerned with some alternative 'models of pedagogy' that might be used in physical education. It is quite likely these (or some) have been a part of initial teacher education and/or induction. For the models selected research has demonstrated positive outcomes for pupils. The models seek to promote teaching which is more student-centred, where pupils take greater responsibility for their and other's learning and the teacher acts in a facilitation role (TLRP, 2007; Rovegno, 2008). Given space this chapter cannot cover the vast range of models appropriate for physical education. Further sources are available which extend the review beyond that presented here (e.g. Metzler, 2000).

Some Definitions

Tinning (2008) argues the term 'pedagogy' is both complex, with several meanings and a number of synonyms. Siedentop (1991) considers pedagogy '. . . as the skilful arrangement of an environment in such a way that students acquire specifically intended learnings. Pedagogy links teachers' actions with students' outcomes' (p. 7). This will be the definition used in this chapter.

Joyce and Showers (1980) viewed an instructional model as '. . . a plan or pattern that can be used to shape curriculums (long-term courses of studies), to design instructional materials, and to guide instruction in the classroom and other settings' (p. 1). A pedagogical model takes a long-term view of instruction with interest in planning, teaching and assessment of learning. Figure 9.1 summarizes some ways in which instructional models might be arranged (a continuum, as a spectrum, in groups).

Alternative Models of Pedagogy

This chapter is designed to help teachers think differently about and expand their repertoire of teaching approaches. The models in this chapter illustrate; greater pupil-to-pupil social interaction, increased pupil decision-making, a fostering of opportunities for peer teaching,

Rink (2001)	Direct ---------------------- Indirect	*Direct*: teacher-centred, content as parts, taught in a step-wise manner *Indirect*: student-centred, holistic
Mosston and Ashworth (2002)	Command --------------- Self-teach	Nine teaching styles on a spectrum based around decision-making
Joyce, Calhoun and Showers (2003)	Behavioural systems family ---------- --- --- ---	– teacher-directed, orderly and task oriented
	Social family ------------------------------ --- ---------------------------------------	– people work together for individual and group growth
	Information processing family	– higher order thinking, solving authentic problems

Figure 9.1 Ways of viewing instruction.

increased inter-dependency and self-reliance. It is hoped the descriptions and research evidence offer some encouragement that a 'shift' to one/some of the models outlined is possible. For example, in one study student teachers were able to transfer and sustain interest in Sport Education [one model presented in this chapter] from initial teacher education to the first few years of teaching. A shared culture of support for innovation from both within the physical education department and from induction tutors/mentors aided this transfer (Curtner-Smith et al., 2008).

> **Reflection**
>
> Identify some factors that might inhibit efforts by teachers to innovate within the Physical Education curriculum in a school. Propose some strategies that might seek to overcome these factors.

In wishing to identify some potential connections between the individual models, Figure 9.2 offers a 'diagrammatic' setting out relationships between and developments of some of these models.

Sport Education and Variants

Sport Education was developed by Daryl Siedentop. Siedentop's (1994) rationale for Sport Education is captured in the following quotation where he claims sport teaching in physical education has typically been decontextualized, leading to an incomplete learning experience:

> Skills are taught in isolation rather than as part of the natural context of executing strategy in game-like situations. The rituals, values and traditions of a sport that give it meaning are seldom

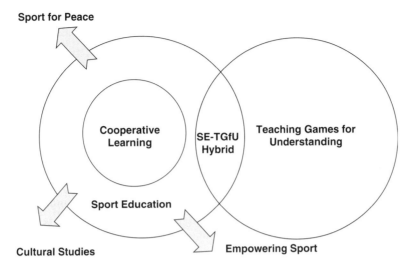

Figure 9.2 Model relationship and development.

mentioned, let alone taught in ways that students can experience them. The affiliation with a team or group that provides the context for personal growth and responsibility in sport is noticeably absent in physical education. The ebb and flow of a sport season is seldom captured in a short-term sport instruction unit. It becomes clear that, too often, physical education teachers only isolated sport skills and less than meaningful games. Students are not educated in sport. (Siedentop, 1994, pp. 7–8)

Given this critique, Sport Education was essentially designed to offer learners an inclusive, positive and enjoyable sport experience to '. . . educate students to be players in the fullest sense and to help them develop as competent, literate, and enthusiastic sportspeople' (Siedentop, 1994, p. 4). By this a competent sportsperson is one who has adequate skill and strategic competence to participate meaningfully within a practice and/or game. A literate sportsperson is cognizant of the particular rules, traditions, and rituals that give sport its unique meaning and who is also sufficiently informed to be able to discern between appropriate and inappropriate sport-related behaviour. Finally, Siedentop deemed an enthusiastic sportsperson as one who advocates for the preservation and development of the wider sporting cultures (Siedentop, 1994).

The fullest sense requires units of work in Sport Education to foreground educationally worthwhile outcomes and include authentic 'sport-simulated' in-class experiences within a framework comprising the essential features that resemble bona fide sport. These features are;

- activities are presented in a **seasonal format** extending units of work beyond the more traditional 4–6 week blocks to, in some instances, up to 18–20 sessions;

- **affiliation**: small-sided groups/teams are established and stay together for the duration of season(s);
- **formal competition** is included through modified arrangements in team size, rules and equipment (e.g. 2vs2) using a combination of student-led and teacher-led practice;
- **records** are kept, which might include league points for win-losses, fair play, supporting others etc.;
- seasons conclude with a **culminating event** resembling what might be seen in major sporting occasions; and
- **festivity** is emphasized through the use of team names, team uniforms, banners and so on.

In addition to being a player, pupils adopt team-based roles and responsibilities that might include captain, coach, equipment manager, timer or umpire. These roles support the gradual shift in pedagogy across a season from teacher-directed to more pupil centred instruction. Work on teams becomes increasingly planned and undertaken by pupils fulfilling these roles. Pupils work co-operatively and their leadership obligations support the managerial/organizational and instructional elements of the sport experience. As teams work towards the formal and culminating competitions they earn a range of points/rewards related to win/losses, sport-like behaviour, performance as an official etc.

Research on Sport Education offers considerable support for this instructional model from both pupils across educational stages and their teachers. The reader is encouraged to access some extensive reviews of this literature (see Wallhead and O'Sullivan, 2005; Kinchin, 2006). Interest in Sport Education has also led to development of some variants. Each aims to capitalize on '... social structures within the complex teaching learning environment that promise the possibility of better learning and social experiences for all learners...' (Rovegno, 2008, p. 94) and evidence from research in schools has been largely positive. Ennis (1999) integrated conflict resolution with the essential curricular features of Sport Education to develop a model termed '*Sport for Peace*'. This model extends Sport Education to accommodate both a concern for and care for others and fosters the development of self and social responsibility. Sport for Peace places emphasis upon developing a pupil's ability to negotiate and compromise in response to conflict. O'Sullivan and Kinchin (in press) outline an integrated practical and theoretical investigation of sport/physical activity by adopting Sport Education in concert with issues of social justice. Known as '*Cultural Studies Curriculum in Physical Activity and Sport*' this approach aims to secure meaningful connections between school-based physical education (as a function of Sport Education) and the provision for sport and physical activity in local, community and national contexts. Acknowledging Siedentop's (1995) recommendation that physical education develop learners who are critical consumers of sport and physical activity, Cultural Studies promotes individual and team-based opportunities to present and defend ideas on social justice through a range of mechanisms including journals, class discussions and team projects. Kinchin and O'Sullivan (2003) reported a number of positive features and pupils saw relevance in discussing issues of gender, sport media and body image. Hastie and Curtner-Smith (2006) successfully field-tested a *hybrid* of Sport Education with Teaching Games for Understanding (TGfU, which is considered in more detail in this chapter) by integrating an emphasis upon developing pupils' tactical and strategic capabilities within the structural elements of Sport Education. Hastie and Buchanan (2000) described how the teaching of personal and social responsibility (see Hellison, 1995) was amalgamated with Sport Education combining responsible role positions and the development of leadership. Termed *Empowering Sport* this model foregrounds fair play while learners engage themselves and others in physical activity exploring the inter-relationship of sport skill and social responsibility. The reader is encouraged to access some of these sources to learn how each might be an ingredient of a physical education programme.

Co-operative Learning

Co-operative learning is an umbrella term that refers to '…a variety of educational approaches involving joint intellectual effort by students, or students and teachers together' (Smith and MacGregor, 1992, p. 10). As was evident in the previous section, co-operative learning is an integral feature of Sport Education in that over time it develops opportunities for pupils to work in teams to ensure all members have mastered an objective. Co-operative learning fits with some current conceptions of learning as a social, cultural and interpersonal process (see TLRP, 2007) and the benefits of this instructional model are many. Learners work together purposefully and actively in small groups to enhance their own and others' learning. Slavin (1983a; 1995) highlights the body of research which has documented; (a) the use of this model to both improve both pupil achievement and social and affective outcomes; (b) helping pupils integrate their knowledge and then apply skills they have learned to other contexts, and (c) how co-operative learning has been found to positively impact social relations with pupils from a range of ethnic backgrounds and also those included within regular classrooms. Co-operative learning has also been successful is helping some children learn to manage conflict (Johnson et al., 1997).

Like Sport Education, co-operative learning places the student at the centre of the learning process in small-sized heterogeneous groups. Two features of co-operative learning exist: positive interdependence and individual accountability (Sharan, 1994). Positive interdependence means the group can only succeed if every member helps, invests in and supports each group-member to complete the task and each individual is therefore held accountable for their share of the work.

Summaries of research evidence on the effectiveness of co-operative learning in classrooms are available (see Johnson and Johnson, 1990; Slavin, 1995). Co-operative learning can promote student academic achievement and the development of many social and interpersonal skills (Slavin, 1983b; Cohen, 1994; Abrami et al., 1995) where emphasis is placed upon students working with each other to complete tasks that are normally set by the teacher, who now acts as a facilitator of learning. Positive interaction is expected and a number of social and affective outcomes have been reported such as improved inter-dependency, self-esteem, and group collaboration. Research has found that teachers feel more successful when using co-operative learning methods, because it affords them opportunities to reach many more students and engage them in learning (Sharan, 1994).

Research has investigated the use of co-operative learning in both primary and secondary physical education (e.g. Dyson, 2001; Polvi and Telama, 2000). This research details the positive influence of co-operative learning on social enhancement, pupil responsibility, performance of motor skill and the promotion of positive verbal interaction.

Teaching Games for Understanding

The roots of this model can be traced back to the work of Bunker, Almond and Thorpe in the early 1980s (e.g. Bunker and Thorpe, 1982; Thorpe et al. 1986). The section on Sport Education made mention of Siedentop's critique of incomplete sport-learning experiences evident in some physical education lessons. Researchers here observed much of the teaching of games was focused on skill/technique development in highly teacher-centred environments with minimal time for game-play. In lessons where game-play followed skill and drill work, limited tactical awareness in learners was evident and skill/technique learned in earlier parts of the lesson rarely transferred to situations when pupils were 'playing the game'. TGfU was developed as a model to not only promote improvement of tactics and strategy but to do so alongside skill development.

Key to TGfU is the use of modified game-like situations designed to meet specific developmental stages of pupils and include adjustments to equipment, rules and area of play – what many physical education teachers might term as 'conditions'. The learning tasks are set in a way to simulate game-contexts and which pose authentic tactical and strategic problems for pupils to solve in their own way through problem-solving and guided study styles of teaching. Such modifications are intended to help learners develop better game competence and decision making.

Teachers using TGfU see the language of lesson goals shifting from performance of a specific skill or technique to solving particular tactical problems such as 'how to create space in attack in football' (see Griffin et al., 1997). Teachers create the conditions for pupils to confront and then attempt to solve such tactical dilemmas employing a range of possible solutions and being facilitated by careful questioning. Opportunities are also presented enabling pupils to practice the key skills inherent within the initial modified activity.

Reflection

Reflect upon the implications of TGfU for the use of high quality questions in lessons with your pupils. What types of questions would be suitable for your learners when experiencing this approach?

Metzler (2000) captures the very essence of TGfU, stating; 'The emphasis is on the development of tactical knowledge that facilitates skill applications in smaller versions of the game so that the student can apply that learning in the full version . . .' (p. 340). Games, given their common tactical problems are classified into invasion, target, fielding run/score and net/wall. The relationship between these categories, in terms of tactical problems, offers opportunity for pupils to transfer performance across the categories. For example, there are likely to be key tactical similarities between table tennis, tennis and badminton or between football, hockey and Ultimate Frisbee.

Like other models presented in this chapter, the literature includes research highlighting the strength of TGfU and its desirability to support the teaching of games and increase student's ability to play games (e.g. French et al., 1996; Turner and Martinek, 1999; Light, 2002). Whilst some have commented on the challenge to some teachers in terms of content knowledge, studies exist where pupils have expressed a preference to learn within the TGfU framework compared to previous time in physical education (e.g. Griffin et al., 1995).

Sequencing the Models

This chapter has illustrated some alternative models appropriate for teaching and learning in physical education. A teacher might be in a position to consider not only the place of these models within their curriculum but perhaps the sequence in which pupils are exposed to these models and their intended outcomes. There is potential for a number of these models to collectively offer an educationally rich and engaging experience reaped with a range of rewards as a function of participation. Figure 9.2 offers one example of how models might be sequenced to form a route or pathway through a curriculum or particular period within a curriculum.

Reflection

A key characteristic of this sequence is the introduction and progressive development of group-based learning and the establishment of micro-learning communities which persist over a sustained period of time. To what extent do you support such a characteristic and what might be the merits and concerns of a curriculum sequenced within Figure 9.3?

Conclusion

This chapter has attempted to outline a number of pedagogical models appropriate for physical education teaching and has both highlighted where research has demonstrated positive outcomes for pupils and where practical materials/resources might be located. In physical education we are fortunate to have a rich array of research-informed choices

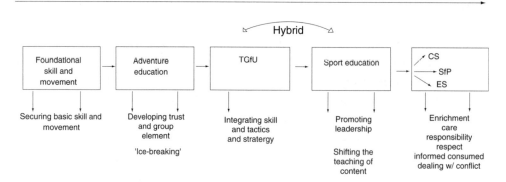

Figure 9.3 Sequencing models.

to assist in the planning of curriculum within schools and which meet pupils' expectations for learning in class. It is hoped the reader might consider one/some of these approaches.

Learning More

Sources to assist in the planning and implementation of Sport Education are available (e.g. Hastie and Kinchin, 2004; Siedentop et al., 2007). Some texts have been written for specific use of co-operative learning in physical education (Grineski, 1996; Kirchner, 2005). Some TGfU sources are available for those interested in putting this instructional approach into practice (e.g. Griffin et al., 1997; Mitchell et al., 2003).

References

Abrami, P.C., Poulson, C. and Chambers, B. (2004) Teacher motivation to implement an educational innovation: Factors differentiating users and non-users of cooperative learning, *Educational Psychology*, 24(2), pp. 201–214.

Bunker, D. and Thorpe, R. (1982) A model for the teaching of games in the secondary school, *Bulletin of Physical Education*, 10, pp. 9–16.

Byra, M. (2006) Teaching styles and inclusive pedagogies (pp. 449–466). In D. Kirk, D. Macdonald and M. O'Sullivan (eds), *The Handbook of Physical Education*. London: Sage.

Capel, S. and Blair, R. (2007) Making physical education relevant: increasing the impact of initial teacher training, *London Review of Education*, 5(1), pp. 15–34.

Cohen, E.G. (1994) *Designing Groupwork: Strategies for the Heterogeneous Classroom*. Second edition. New York: Teachers College Press.

Curtner-Smith, M.D. (1999) The more things change the more they stay the same: factors influencing teachers' interpretations and delivery of National Curriculum Physical Education, *Sport, Education and Society*, 4(1), pp. 75–97.

Curtner-Smith, M.D., Hastie, P.A. and Kinchin. G.D. (2008) Influence of occupational socialization on beginning teachers' interpretation and delivery of sport education, *Sport, Education and Society*, 13(1), pp. 97–117.

Dyson, B. (2001) Cooperative learning in an elementary physical education program, *Journal of Teaching in Physical Education*, 20, pp. 264–281.

Ennis, C.D. (1996) Students' experiences in sport-based physical education: more than apologies are necessary, *Quest*, 48, pp. 453–456.

—(1999) Creating a culturally relevant curriculum for disengaged girls, *Sport, Education and Society*, 4(1), pp. 31–50.

—(2000) Canaries in the coalmine: responding to disengaged students using a theme-based curricula, *Quest*, 52, pp. 119–130.

French, K.E., Werner, P.H., Rink, J.E., Taylor, K. and Hussey, K. (1996) The effects of a 3-week unit of tactical, skill or combined tactical and skill instruction on badminton performance of ninth grade students, *Journal of Teaching in Physical Education*, 15, pp. 418–438.

Green, K. (1998) Philosophies, ideologies and the practice of physical education. *Sport, Education and Society*, 3, pp. 125–143.

—(2008) *Understanding Physical Education*. London: Sage.

Griffin, L.L., Oslin, J.L. and Mitchell, S.A. (1995) An analysis of two institutional approaches to teaching net games, *Research Quarterly for Exercise and Sport*, 66 (Suppl.), pp. 65–66.

Griffin, L.L., Mitchell, S.A. and Oslin, J.L. (1997) *Teaching Sport Concepts and Skills: a Tactical Games Approach*. Champaign, IL: Human Kinetics.

Grineski, S. (1996) *Cooperative Learning in Physical Education*. Champaign, IL: Human Kinetics.

Hastie, P.A. and Buchanan, A.M. (2000) Teaching responsibility through sport education: prospects for a coalition, *Research Quarterly for Exercise and Sport*, 71, pp. 25–35.

Hastie, P.A. and Curtner-Smith, M.D. (2006) Influence of a hybrid Sport Education: Teaching Games for Understanding unit on one teacher and his students, *Physical Education and Sport Pedagogy*, 11, pp. 1–27.

Hastie, P.A. and Kinchin. G.D. (2004) Design a season of sport education, *British Journal of Teaching Physical Education*, 35(1), pp. 14–18.

Hellison, D. (1995) *Teaching Responsibility through Physical Activity*. Champaign, IL: Human Kinetics.

Johnson, D. and Johnson, R. (1990) Cooperative learning and achievement (pp. 173–202). In S. Sharan (ed.), *Cooperative Learning: Theory and Research*. New York: Praeger.

Johnson, D., Johnson, R., Dudley, B., Mitchell, J. and Fredrickson, J. (1997) The impact of conflict resolution training on middle school students, *The Journal of Social Psychology*, 137, pp. 11–21.

Joyce, B., Calhoun, E. and Hopkins, D. (2003) *Models of Teaching, Tools for Learning*. Buckingham: Open University Press.

Joyce. B. and Showers, B. (1980) Improving in-service training: The messages of research, *Educational Leadership*, 37(5), pp. 379–385.

Kinchin, G.D. (2006) Sport Education: a view of the research (pp. 596–609). In D. Kirk, D. Macdonald and M. O'Sullivan (eds), *The Handbook of Physical Education*. London: Sage.

Kinchin, G.D., and O'Sullivan, M. (2003) Incidences of student support for and resistance to a curricular innovation in high school physical education, *Journal of Teaching in Physical Education*, 22(3), pp. 245–260.

Kirk, D. (2005) Model-based teaching and assessment in physical education: The tactical games model (pp.128–142). In K. Green and K. Hardman (eds), *Physical Education: Essential Issues*. London: Sage.

Kircher, G. (2005) *Towards Cooperative Learning in Elementary School Physical Education*. Springfield, IL: Charles C Thomas Publisher Ltd.

Light, R. (2002) Engaging the body in learning: Promoting cognition in games through TGfU. *ACHPER Healthy Lifestyles Journal*, 49(2), pp. 23–26.

Metzler, M. (2000) *Instructional Models for Physical Education*. Boston, MA: Allyn and Bacon.

Mitchell, S.A., Oslin, J.L. and Griffin, L.L. (2003) *Sport Foundations for Elementary Physical Education: A Tactical Games Approach*. Champaign, IL: Human Kinetics.

Mosston, M. and Ashworth, S. (2002) *Teaching Physical Educatio*. Fifth edition. San Francisco, CA: Benjamin Cummings.

O'Sullivan, M. and Kinchin, G.D. (in press) Cultural Studies Curriculum in Sport and Physical Activity. In J. Lund and D. Tannehill (eds), *Standards-Based Physical Education Curriculum Development*. Second edition. Sudbury, MA: Jones and Bartlett Publishers.

Polvi, S. and Telama, R. (2000) The use of co-operative learning as a social enhancer in physical education, *Scandinavian Journal of Educational Research*, 44(1), 105–115.

Rink, J.E. (2001) Investigating the assumptions of pedagogy, *Journal of Teaching in Physical Education*, 20, pp. 112–128.

Rovegno, I. (2008) Learning and instruction in social, cultural environments: Promising research agendas, *Quest*, 60, pp. 84–104.

Sharan, S. (ed.) (1994) *Handbook of Cooperative Learning Methods*. Westport, CT: Greenwood Press.

Siedentop, D. (1991) *Developing Teaching Skills in Physical Education*. Third edition. Mountain View, CA: Mayfield Publishing Company.

—(1994) *Sport Education*. Champaign, IL: Human Kinetics.

—(1995) Improving sport education. *ACHPER Healthy Lifestyles Journal*, 42(4), pp. 22–23.

Siedentop, D., Hastie, P.A. and van der Mars, H. (2007) *The Complete Guide to Sport Education*. Champaign, IL: Human Kinetics.

Slavin, R.E. (1983a) When does cooperative learning increase student achievement? *Psychological Bulletin*, 94, pp. 429–445.

—(1983b) *Cooperative Learning*. New York: Longman.

—(1995) *Cooperative Learning: Theory, Research, and Practice*. Second edition. Boston, MA: Allyn and Bacon.

Smith, B.L. and MacGregor, J.T. (1992) What is collaborative learning? (pp. 9–22). In A. Goodsell, M. Maher and V. Tinto (eds), *Collaborative Learning: A Sourcebook for Higher Education*. University Park, PA: National Center on Postsecondary Teaching, Learning and Assessment.

Thorpe, R., Bunker, D. and Almond, L. (1986) *Rethinking Games Teaching*. Loughborough: Loughborough University.

Teaching and Learning Research Programme (TLRP) (2007) *Principles into Practice: A Teacher's Guide to Research Evidence on Teaching and Learning*. London: TLRP.

Tinning, R. (2008) Pedagogy, sport pedagogy and the field of kinesiology, *Quest*, 60, pp. 405–424.

Turner, A. and Martinek, T. (1999) An investigation into teaching games for understanding: effects on skill, knowledge and game play, *Research Quarterly for Exercise and Sport*, 70(3), pp. 286–296.

Wallhead, T. and O'Sullivan, M. (2005) Sport Education: physical education for the new millennium? *Physical Education and Sport Pedagogy*, 10(2), pp. 181–210.

Using ICT to Enhance Learning in Physical Education

10

Graham Parton and Matthew Light

Technology has the potential to enhance and support pupils' learning. The popularity and use of new technology amongst pupils opens up new possibilities for physical education and poses challenges to those looking to utilize information and communication technology in pupils learning. This chapter considers the learning potential of new and existing technologies and offers examples of how they can become an integral part of physical education teaching.

An Integrated Approach to the Use of ICT in Physical Education

ICT and standards

Information and Communication Technology (ICT) as a subject has seen much growth over the last two decades; however, there is little evidence that ICT is revolutionizing teaching and learning (Goodson and Mangan, 1995). Governments around the world have invested heavily in supplying schools with the infrastructure to deliver ICT. ICT education has become a highly politicized agenda (Hennessy et al., 2005) and has developed a 'rhetoric of modernisation' which Leach and Moon (2000) argue has barely touched teaching and learning. One of the main problems with the adoption of ICT into teaching and learning is that in many countries, the focus has been on using ICT to raise standards. Reports carried out in the UK concerning the impact of ICT on standards have been inconclusive. The IMPACT2 report showed that there was little gain in standards between children who used computers frequently and children that do not (Harrison et al., 2002). This is mirrored by research completed in the USA and Australia (Cuban, 1993). He argues that:

> There is no clear, commanding body of evidence that students' sustained use of multimedia machines, the internet, word processing, spreadsheets, and other popular applications has an impact on academic achievement. (p. 3)

The evidence, regarding standards is quite damming and throws doubt on using ICT. However if standards are taken out of the equation, the use of ICT and its role in the learning process looks much brighter.

ICT and learning

It is argued that research should investigate the mechanisms by which children learn with ICT rather than from ICT (Kozma, 1994). That is ICT should be researched within the learning process rather than in isolation. He states that a problem concerning ICT within education is that new technologies are being fitted into old curricula, which were developed prior to their existence. One of the main aims of integrating ICT is the belief that children will gain skills that will equip them when they enter the workforce of the future (Noss and Pachler, 1999).

There is a growing view that ICT should be taught in as an integrated or cross-curricular subject, rather than teaching ICT as a single subject (Reynolds et al., 2003). This means that subjects such as physical education can incorporate ICT to enhance and personalize children's learning. It has been suggested that when ICT is integrated into a curriculum effectively that a change in the learning process occurs (CEO Forum, 1999). These changes are identified as:

- Problem orientated – use of ICT allows authentic investigations which provide a variety of solutions;
- Child-centered – children feel empowered, creating and developing their own investigations;
- Collaborative – investigations involve working together which promotes team work;
- Relevant and productive – ICT has the potential to provide educational experiences which meet the needs of diverse learners. ICT encourages children to become content producers;
- Lifelong – skills used when completing investigations are of benefit in the long term.

The main aims, therefore, of an integrated approach to ICT are:

- To encourage the use of technology to enhance higher order thinking (Kim and Hang, 2003);
- To motivate and challenge learners;
- To encourage problem solving and interrogation of data (Noss and Pachler, 1999);
- To be able to effectively research, evaluate and refine information (Kennewell and Parkinson, 2000);
- To encourage the use of ICT in a project based curriculum, which develops and understanding of the holistic nature of learning (Miller, 1999).

We argue that in order to develop these skills it is important that you integrate ICT into your teaching, where physical education is the context and the use of ICT are the tools used to understand and interpret the data and ideas posed by the context.

Physical education and ICT

Good practice guidelines on the effective use of ICT in physical education lessons are limited and in need of development. However, appropriate planning and evaluation of how technologies are used in lessons is a basic prerequisite of good teaching with technology. Bailey (2001) indicates that decisions about when and when not to use ICT in lessons should be based on whether the use of technologies supports good practice in the subject, relate directly to the learning and teaching objectives of lessons and units of work, and allow users to achieve or learn something more effectively or efficiently. If ICT is to be integrated into lessons it should be done as a natural part of the teaching and learning process and not considered as an add-on to normal teaching.

Teachers therefore need to consider what it is they are trying to achieve, how they are going to organize learning that takes place and how they are achieving their aims. In recent years changes made to school curriculums have indicated a set of learning skills which are important for successful lifelong learning. These skills include being a reflective learner; team worker; creative thinker and an independent and enquiring learner. The inclusion of technologies in physical education has the potential to support pupils in the learning process. This includes empowering learners to construct their own knowledge; develop intellectual and co-operative partnerships amongst pupils; and cater for the wide range of learning styles, rates of learning and interest (MacDonald, 2004).

One possible curriculum model which may be able to effectively incorporate a number of these learning skills is that of Sport Education (Siedentop, 1994). One of the key characteristics of this model is that pupils take on different roles related to the activity beyond that of a player/performer. The range of different roles and responsibilities are designed to maximize links to 'wider learning' in the school. If technologies are to be integrated into pupils learning experiences throughout the school then physical education teachers should plan for to use the full range of ICT equipment available to them. Outlined below (Figure 10.1) is a summary

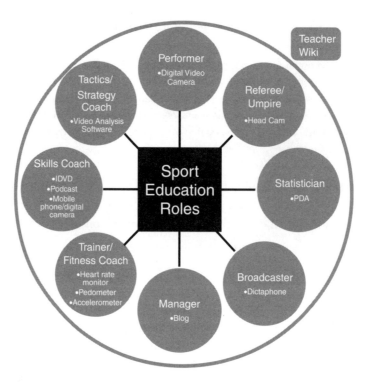

Figure 10.1 An illustration of how different technologies could be employed during a Sport Education season.

of how some ICT equipment may be effectively employed in Sport Education lessons to assist the learning and understanding of different roles (see Chapter 9 for a detailed outline of the Sport Education model).

The challenge for the teacher in this model is how to organize the learning experiences. A shift towards more a pupil-centred pedagogy in this model holds many challenges for both the teacher and pupils. Supporting pupil led learning with ICT requires effective planning and understanding of technologies. An example of how a range of technologies could be used in a basketball Sport Education season is illustrated (Figure 10.2). Much of the collected data can be kept and monitored using a wiki. This would allow the teacher to monitor and assess pupil attainment during the Sport Education season and give feedback and set targets for future progress.

Communication-based Technologies

Wikis, blogs and podcasts (Web 2.0 tools)

In recent years there has been increasing interest from the education community in the use of web-based collaborative software namely wikis, blogs and podcasts (also known as

Role	Technology	Potential Use
Performer	Digital video camera	The performer can view their set shot performance during a game looking at technique or their positioning on the court when using a zone defence.
Referee/Umpire	Head Cam	The referee can review decisions made during a game and the effectiveness of their court positioning.
Statistician	PDA	The statistician can input individual player data onto the spreadsheet during play. Information may include feedback and could relate to free throw and set shot percentages.
Broadcaster	Dictaphone	The broadcaster could give a running commentary during game play and later overlaid onto a video of the game.
Manager/Organizer	Blog	The tournament organizers can communicate information relating to safety, risk assessment and procedures and processes necessary for the smooth running of the event.
Train/Fitness coach	Heart rate monitor Accelerometer	The trainer could use heart rate date to illustrate the effects of different types of training. Also using accelerometers distance travelled during the game can be analysed and linked to specific player training programmes during the season.
Skills coach	Podcasts	Short exemplar videos can be created and shared with the team via a web portal to illustrate teaching cues for different skills such as a jump shot, set shot and lay up shot.
Tactics/Strategy coach	Video analysis software	Game play can be 'tagged' to illustrate examples of man to man defence or the effective use of the fast break.

Figure 10.2 An example of technologies being used during a basketball Sport Education season.

Web 2.0 tools). These tools have considerable potential for addressing the diverse needs of today's learners, by enhancing their learning experiences through customization, personalization, and by providing rich opportunities for networking and collaboration (Bryant, 2006). It is the sociability aspect of these tools which may prove to have the most potential for enhancing education. Boyd (2007) believes that this aspect supports three ingredients or activities that characterize learner-centred instruction, namely: (i) support for conversational interaction; (ii) support for social feedback; and (iii) support for social networks and relationships between people. These 'social software' tools require limited technical skills allowing the user to focus on the information and collaborative tasks. There is evidence from schools to suggest that access to and use of Web 2.0 technologies by secondary-age pupils is already widespread and prolific (Luckin et al., 2008).

Wikis and blogs

The term 'wiki' is derived from the Hawaiian phrase wiki-wiki which means quick. A wiki is a collaborative website whose content can be edited by visitors to the site, allowing users to easily create and edit web pages collaboratively (Chao, 2007).The world's largest and most popular wiki is Wikipedia 'The Free Encyclopedia'. It is a multi language, web-based encyclopedia which encourages online collaboration and interaction by its users. Different wiki providers offer different features but common elements are (a) the ability to create and edit pages, and (b) the ability to compare pages and to track the editing process. This allows the community of users to monitor the changing state of the wiki and discuss the issues which emerge. Wikis can also be used as a source of information and knowledge sharing as well as a tool for learning within a collaborative learning partnership (Parker and Chao, 2007).

Other features allow the teacher to monitor student's participation and receive e-mail prompts when changes or updates have occurred to web pages. This enables them to police student input and edit any unwanted or malicious comments. Users can also incorporate sounds, movies and pictures directly to the wiki. This allows for a collaborative and integrated approach to sharing different media content.

Blogs differ from wikis because individual posting remain the property of individual authors and are unable to be edited by others. The differences between blogs and wikis are subtle but they differ in the way they organize information and in what contributor intend to achieve. In general terms a 'blog' refers to something like an online journal or diary, although their use goes beyond merely recording events or information. They can be written by individuals or collaborative groups with dated entries recorded in reverse chronological order (most recent first). These postings are typically short normally one to three paragraphs of text and may also feature pictures and links to other websites. The dynamic nature of blogs means that postings are often regularly updated. This means readers need to regularly check for new postings. To overcome this blogs can be tracked using RSS (Really Simple Syndication) feeds which alert the reader that new posting have been made without the need to send lots of e-mails. Examples of RSS feeds are numerous in the world of sport regularly informing the reader of breaking news or items of interest (e.g. http://talkingeducationandsport.blogspot.com/).

Reflection

Ask the students to create a wiki or collaborative blog which consists of a resource for physical education-related news and resources. Students can trawl the internet and post the URL of effective resources and other blogs related to teaching and learning in physical education.

Podcasts and vodcasts

Podcasts and vodcasts are audio and video files which are able to be listened/watched anywhere, any time and any place at the convenience of the user. These files are able to be uploaded to a desktop computer or portable media device such as MP3 and MP4 player. Audio files can be created by using a digital Dictaphone, recordable MP3 player or PDA (personal digital assistant). The files are then converted into MP3 format via editing software such as Audacity. The finished work can then be uploaded to a school virtual learning environment or a blog. Vodcasts are recorded using a digital camera or mobile phone and are edited and converted to an MP4 format via computer software. The finished work is then uploaded to a website such as iTunes or MP4 player.

Underpinning pedagogy of Web 2.0 tools

A pedagogical framework for the implementation of these 'social software' tools can be developed by drawing on concepts such as constructivism, social constructivism and communities of practice. The collaborative features of these tools make them suited for co-operative learning environments which can lead to helpful interdependence of group members and individual accountability. Indeed this type of learning has the potential for co-operative groups retaining information for longer than those who work individually (Johnson and Johnson, 1986). Mutual learning can potentially become more powerful if it takes place in a community of practice, that is, people engaged in learning in a shared area of interest. Indeed Lave and Wenger (1991) assert that passive members of a community learn from active members and are gradually brought into an active role in that community. These technologies can be used as a knowledge platform for users to share information, debate ideas and discuss issues.

Many aspects of working with wikis and blogs involve a constructivist approach to learning. They allow pupils to integrate new ideas with prior knowledge to make meaning and enable learning through reflection. An essential part of reflective, constructivist learning is that learners are invited to reflect on their own knowledge and to understand their own learning processes. This can be achieved through traditional means such as essays and project work. However, these technologies allow this reflection to be done collaboratively, moving the learning towards a socially constructed mode of learning.

Practical applications of wikis, blogs and podcasts in physical education

The e-portfolio

At a basic level of use a wiki, blogs and podcasts allow students to post, review and access relevant media by uploading content. This allows teachers and students to work closely together on a topic without the need to necessarily meet together. However, a potentially more powerful use of these learning technologies is when they are integrated to form a record of progress and achievement, that is, a portfolio or e-portfolio. E-portfolios focus on pupils progress and development over time, with regular reflection on progress and achievements made, along with goal setting and self evaluation. To work effectively teachers need to set the parameters of what is to be included in an e-portfolio and clearly indicate the assessment criteria for users. Wikis, blog and podcasts can be used to host content that could be included in an e-portfolio.

Case Study: Project Work

Topic: training programme

The teacher sets up a number of individual wikis for pupils. The content uploaded includes assessment criteria, web links to relevant materials, templates which outline the parameters of the project. Pupils upload written training plans over a period of time which contains data relating to fitness tests and how they have used their knowledge and understanding of principles of training. Pupils can reflect on their training by uploading audio commentary on a podcast and show evidence of safe practice when performing fitness tests or lifting weights with the use of a vodcast. The teacher supports the learning from a distance by reading, annotating and tracking progress via the wiki and by answering pupil questions via their own blog.

Example of Collaborative Working

Topic: sport education

The teacher sets up a number of 'team' wikis for groups of pupils taking part in an athletics sport education season. When pupils are performing their different team roles they upload content to the wiki for use by the team. For example, the tactics/strategy coach can discuss strategies with their teammates about upcoming games; the skills 'coach' can produce a vodcast showing others in the team how to perform skills, with the use of an MP4 player the content could then be used in practical lessons as a reciprocal aid to learning; the team 'reporter/broadcaster' can post a match report allowing team members to add depth and detail about match content. Individual and team statistics can be continuously updated and amended during the season with pages being reviewed by the teacher to review pupil progress over time.

Activity

Ask a group of children to set up a Twitter© (http://twitter.com) page which is based on an area of physical education. Twitter is a social networking site which allows brief statements to be added to a web page. This page could be concerned with the results of a real-time location-based activity. For example:

9.30 a.m. 12 February: Team 2 have found the first clue, what could it mean?
9.45 a.m. 12 February: Team 3 have found the second clue, can we win the whole thing?

This provides the children with a real-time report of what happened and the significant events. This will help with reflecting upon their performance and how other teams worked together to complete the activity. A problem with using social networking tools is their safety and privacy. Analyse the appropriateness of the site before using them with children and find out ways to make the children's experience more private.

Assessment-based Technologies: Motion Capture and Analysis Technologies

What are assessment technologies?

Common feature associated with all motion capture technologies is the ability of the user to take 'in action' clips for future analysis. Another aspect is the accessibility and portability of devices, which allows physical education teachers to use this technology in a wider and more dynamic range of physical activities. The robust construction of many devices like head cams and digital cameras means they can be taken underwater or imaginatively positioned on helmets, handlebars or different parts of the body to offer a range of viewpoints to observe movement. Many cameras allow the user to take single shots or slow motion analysis via functions such as 'multi burst' which slows down the playback and affords the user a chance to review action in greater detail. The popularity of mobile phones among many pupils gives teachers the opportunity to use the camera function of this devise as an easy method of collecting images and short video clips. The added benefit is that little training is required to make the footage accessible. There may be some apprehension about the use of mobile phone with the potential for 'cyber bullying' and the misuse of images. However, if lessons are carefully planned and images of pupils are restricted to their own phones these fears can be effectively managed. Motion analysis technologies can be used to review footage of performances using the screen of a digital camera and DVD players or stored and manipulated with specific video analysis software packages.

Practical uses of assessment technologies

Teachers need to be able to assess pupil's skills, knowledge and understanding in a range of activities. Involving pupils in the process of assessment can significantly contribute to their own understanding (Bailey, 2001). Using a range of technologies such as digital cameras and video analysis packages allows pupils to be actively involved in their own learning. The potential uses of these technologies for pupils includes analysing their own and others techniques and performances. This could be illustrated by asking pupils to view footage of a skill from different angles so greater detail of performances is able to be seen. Then by using camera functions such 'multi-burst' or a software package the footage can be viewed as a still picture or in slow motion enabling pupils to prioritize and make decisions to bring about improved performance. Portable technologies such as interactive DVD players have been successfully used in lessons as a visual guide of the correct technical model for skill development (Clarke and Barton, 2007). Footage of skills in different areas of activity include swimming strokes, gymnastics vaults, dance motifs, athletics throws, tennis serves etc.

Video analysis packages allow pupils to review in detail episodes of activity. This footage has the potential to increase pupil knowledge and understanding of how skills are applied and may help them refine and adapt their tactics, strategies and compositional ideas more effectively. Some software packages allow the user to 'tag' events which occur enabling a series of movie clips to be compiled illustrating specific events for pupils and teachers to focus upon. Practical examples include reviewing the effectiveness of routes taken after orienteering using footage from a head cam; evaluating the composition of an artistic dance routine or gymnastics sequence (e.g. trampolining routine); a discussion of planned tactics and strategies in games activities and the effective use of pacing in athletics and swimming races.

Health-related Technologies: Exergaming (or 'exertainment')

Public health bodies across the world continue to report that children are leading increasingly more sedentary lifestyles. Physical education's contribution to pupil's health lies in its ability to help them make informed choices about adopting healthy and active lifestyles. The use of active video gaming (so called 'exergaming' or 'exertainment') technology in promoting positive health-related behaviours offers teachers the opportunity capitalize on the popularity of video games. Examples include:

- *Dance Dance Revolution (DDR)* which involves players moving to music and stepping on dance pads which are connected to a games console. Arrows that flash on the TV screen cue players when to take steps; higher scores are awarded when players' steps match the tempo of the flashing arrows.

- *Nintendo, Wii Sports* and *Wii Fit* which have a traditional game controller with buttons but the addition of an accelerometer and infrared sensors to detect the controller's position in and movement through three-dimensional space. The *Wii Fit* also has a balance board to control gaming interaction.

A review of research through 2006 indicates that video games have the potential to promote positive health-related behaviour change. Using social cognitive theory as a model of learning for behaviour change, Baranowski et al. (2008) point out that the process involves attention, retention, production and motivation. Games add an element of fun, an aspect of intrinsic motivation, thereby enhancing behaviour change through enhanced motivation.

Users of *DDR* have shown that its use has the potential to meet daily cardio-respiratory requirements (Tan et al., 2002) and maybe of benefit to vulnerable groups indicating that overweight children burned more calories than non-overweight children (Unnithan et al., 2006). Those playing *Wii Sports* used more energy than when playing sedentary video games but not as much energy as playing 'real' sports (Graves et al., 2007). Besides the physiological benefits of using 'exergames' their use in physical education classes have shown positive results with pupils indicating improved self-concept, social skills and enthusiasm towards sports, fitness and dance (Sashek, 2004).

Traditional Health-related Technologies

In recent years there has been a growth in the range and scope of technologies which are able to record, analyse and interpret data relating to fitness and health. Many of these devises like treadmills, rowing machines and cross trainers are in regular use in many schools. They have many functions including allowing the user to plan and individualize their own programmes. Users are able to select the difficulty of the task by changing the incline on treadmills or the resistance on a bike or cross trainer. Data such as distance covered, average speed and calories burnt can then be used to talk about the principles of training or aspect of health related to energy expenditure.

The use of recording devices to collect data in physical education is well established. Heart rate monitors, blood pressure monitors, electric peak flow meters and pedometers are useful in enabling pupils to interpret date relating to the effects of exercise on the body. Information from heart rate monitors can be easily sent to laptops via USB or Bluetooth and a data base of peak flow readings can be directly uploaded to a spread sheet for analysis. Pedometers and accelerometers measure distance travelled and devices like the Nike+ system are able to record with some accuracy the pace and time taken to complete a course. The device is placed inside a Nike trainer or between the laces of other training shoes. With the inclusion of an IPod the accelerometer tracks distance, speed, and time-taken and gives you an audible read-out of your present pace and time taken. Once completed the data can then be uploaded to the Nike+ website to show a graph of their speed, distance and time taken to complete the activity (see Figure 10.3).

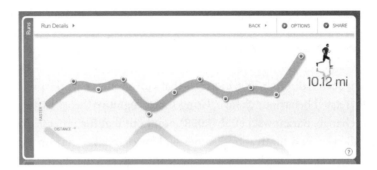

Figure 10.3 Nike+ running chart (www.nikeplus.nike.com).

Reflection

Set up a circuit consisting of different cardiovascular exercises. Fit accelerometers onto the children's trainers. Once the children have completed the exercises, download the data to a computer and analyse the data with the children. Ask questions such as: How could you improve your time with this exercise? Could you improve your technique and what effect would this have on the data?

The benefits to pupils of these technologies are that they are able to have accurate measurements of the intensity of their exercise and information which helps them to have a visual representation of concepts such as oxygen uptake, training zones, the effects steady rate exercise on heart rate and comparison of different types of training on aerobic and anaerobic exercise. They also allow pupils to set their own targets which can be constantly assessed and updated by the pupil and as a measure of progress by teachers.

Location-based Technologies

What is location-based technology?

Global Positioning System (GPS) is a technology which utilizes a system of satellites and computers which determine the latitude and longitude of a receiver. It does this by calculating the time difference that the signal from the satellites take to reach the receiver. There are many types of receiver available for schools to use. The most popular are hand-held products from Garmin and are relatively inexpensive. Some mobile phones such as Nokia, HTC and the Apple iPhone have GPS. Garmin also have watches which contain GPS which are ultra-portable and excellent for tracking activities.

Practical uses of location-based technology

Geocaching is becoming a popular global activity. The idea behind Geocaching is to hide a plastic box which contains prizes or caches in a certain location which has been recorded by a GPS receiver. This location is then uploaded to a website along with clues and the title of the cache. Many caches are now hidden all over the world, some which are easier to find than others! One of the highest caches being found at Mount Everest's base camp. These caches are managed from a central website, http://geocaching.com. Registration is free but it is required to view the latitude and longitude of the caches.

Geocaching fits very nicely into the area of orienteering as checkpoints can be setup around a school's grounds and then uploaded to the website for the children to use using portable computers such as netbooks or PDA's. A clue can be hidden at each checkpoint which guides them to the next location's latitude and longitude. Once all checkpoints have been found the final checkpoint can be a prize or a code which needs to be deciphered. Children can also use digital cameras or mobile phones to record the checkpoints and then bring them back for evidence. To increase the fitness requirement the children could run or jog between the checkpoints.

A valuable aspect of using GPS receivers is that they record real-time data of the children's activity. This can then be downloaded to Google Maps (see Figure 10.4). This then gives a view of the trail overlaid by satellite images of the terrain. A typical example is shown below:

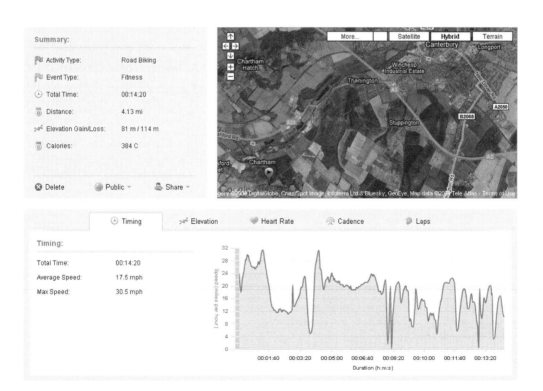

Figure 10.4 Activity results page ©Garmin Connect.

Once the children are experienced in geocaching, they can start to design their own or look on the website for local caches. Designing a cache is relatively easy and it is free to upload them once they have been completed. In this way the children can share their geocaches with their class friends. A very recent development in location-based technology is location-based social gaming. Software can be downloaded to Java-based mobile phones which then use GPS and the mobile internet to allow teams of players to search for waypoints within a specified location. The object of the game is for teams to capture as many waypoints as possible to win the game. Location-based gaming is very new and one of the first games to be published was Torality. Further information can be found at http:// tourality.com/

What is the learning potential for location-based technologies?

GPS technology has the power to track a child's movement, speed and distance. This allows children to guide themselves to a specific predetermined space. This type of guided walking or jogging promotes life-long fitness as it is both fun and demanding physically. The myriad of immediate data gathered by these activities can be used to evaluate their performance when searching for the caches, this data can also be used to plan for ways they could improve their performance and skills. These activities also promote collaboration amongst the geo-caching team, as success is increased if the children work as a team and solve problems together. Problem-solving is key to geocaching as it allows a child-centred approach to the activity. Resilience is also an attitude which is promoted as it takes patience to look for the cache and solve the clues along the way. Motivation is also increased by using this technology as the activity is challenging and exciting.

Reflection

1. Using a location-based game such as *Tourality*, set up waypoints around the school playground and fields. Organize the children into teams with a GPS-assisted mobile phone and set them off. First team to capture all of the waypoints wins. Once the game is finished the data from the game such as time taken, fastest capture, time between waypoints can be used to reflect upon the game and the children's performance.
2. Ask the children to plan and develop their own geocache within the school grounds. This can consist of one cache or a series of minicaches which give a clue to the next one until they orientate to the final cache.

Conclusion

This chapter has considered the learning potential of new and existing technologies and has offered examples of how they can become an integral part of physical education teaching. It has been argued that there needs to be a change in how ICT is used in education as it has been shown that ICT does not have a significant effect on standards. Using the principles of sport education it can be seen that ICT can be integrated effectively in physical education as a learning tool. The use of ICT as a learning tool gives a much wider perspective on the use of technology and the learning benefits it can bring for children. These are exciting times for physical education and ICT as many new technologies are emerging, such as location-based technologies, which bring a more creative and problem-orientated perspective on learning.

Learning More

Sources to assist in the planning and implementation of ICT in physical education are available (Leith and Hall, 2001; Castelli and Fiorentino, 2008). Reports illustrating the use of ICT in physical education and uptake and impact of ICT in schools have been written (Wood, 2005; Condie and Munroe, 2007; Smith et al., 2008). Some resources are available for those interested in the pedagogy of e-learning (Beetham and Sharpe, 2007) and the implementation of Web 2.0 technologies in the classroom (Richardson, 2008).

References

Bailey, R.P. (2001) *Teaching Physical Education: A Handbook for Primary and Secondary School Teachers*. London: Routledge.

Baranowski, T., Buday, R., Thompson, D. and Baranowski, J. (2008) Playing for real – Video games and stories for health-related behavior change, *American Journal of Preventive Medicine*, 34(1), pp. 74–82.

Beetham, H. and Sharpe, R. (2007) *Rethinking Pedagogy for a Digital Age: Designing and Delivering E-learning*. London: Routledge.

Boyd, D. (2007) The significance of social software. In T.N. Burg and J. Schmidt (eds), *BlogTalks Reloaded: Social Software Research and Cases*. Norderstedt, Germany: Books on Demand.

Bryant, T. (2006) Social software in academia, *EDUCAUSE Quarterly*, 29(2), pp. 61–64.

Castelli, D.M. and Fiorentino L.H. (2008) *Physical Education Technology Playbook*. Champaign, IL: Human Kinetics.

CEO Forum (1999) Professional development: a link to better learning. http://www.ceoforum.org/reports.cfm?RID=2.

Clarke, N. and Barton, G. (2007) A novel teaching and learning approach for physical education – case study, *Physical Education Matters*, 2(2), pp. 18–19.

Condie, R. and Munroe, B. (2007) *The Impact of ICT in Schools: A Landscape Review*. Coventry: British Educational Communications and Technology Agency.

Cuban, L. (1993) Computers meet classroom: classroom wins, *Teachers' College Record*, 95(2), pp. 185–210.

Goodson, I.F. and Mangan, J.M. (1995) Developing a collaborative research strategy with teachers for the study of classroom computing, *Journal of Information Technology for Teacher Education*, 4(3), pp. 269–286.

Graves, L., Stratton, G., Ridgers, N.D. and Cable, N.T. (2007) Comparison of energy expenditure in adolescents when playing new generation and sedentary computer games: cross sectional study, *British Medical Journal*, 335(7633), pp. 1282–1284.

Hall, A. and Leigh, J. (2001) *ICT in Physical Education*. Cambridge: Pearson Publishing.

Harrison, C., Comber, C., Fisher, T., Haw, K., Lewin, C., Linzer, E., McFarlane, A., Mavers, D., Scrimshaw, P., Somekh, B. and Watling, R. (2002) *ImpaCT2: The Impact of Information and Communication Technologies on Pupil Learning and Attainment*. Coventry: British Educational Communications and Technology Agency.

Hennessy, S., Ruthven, K. and Brindley, S. (2005) Teacher perspectives on integrating ICT into subject teaching: commitment, constraints, caution and change, *Journal of Curriculum Studies*, 37(2), pp. 155–192.

Kennewell, S. and Parkinson, J. (2000) *Developing the ICT-capable School*. London: Routledge.

Kim, C. and Hang, D. (2003) An activity theory approach to research of ICT integration in Singapore schools, *Computers and Education*, 41(1), pp. 49–63.

Kozma, R.B. (1994) Will media influence learning? Reframing the debate, *Educational Technology Research and Development*, 42(2), pp. 7–19.

Lave, J. and Wenger, E. (1991) *Situated Learning: Legitimate Peripheral Participation*. Cambridge: Cambridge University Press.

Leach, J. and Moon, B. (2000) Pedagogy, information and communications technology and teachers' professional knowledge, *Curriculum Journal*, 11(3), pp. 385–404.

Luckin, R., Logan, K., Clark, W., Graber, R., Oliver, M. and Mee, A. (2008) *Learners' Use of Web 2.0 Technologies in and out of School in Key Stages 3 and 4*. Coventry: British Educational Communications and Technology Agency.

Macdonald, D. (2004) Understanding learning in physical education (pp. 16–31). In J.D. Wright, D. Macdonald and L. Burrow (eds), *Critical Inquiry and Problem Solving in Physical Education*. London: Routledge.

Miller, J. (1999) Making connections through holistic learning, *Educational Leadership*, 56(4), pp. 46–48.

Noss, R. and Pachler, N. (1999) The challenge of new technologies: doing old things in a new way, or doing new things? (pp. 195–211). In P. Mortimore (ed.), *Understanding Pedagogy and Its Impact on Learning*. London: Paul Chapman.

Parker, K.R. and Chao, J.T. (2007) Wiki as a tool, *Interdisciplinary Journal of Knowledge and Learning Objects*, 3, pp. 57–72.

Reynolds, D., Treharne, D. and Tripp, H. (2003) ICT – the hopes and the reality, *British Journal of Educational Technology*, 34(2), pp. 151–167.

Richardson, W. (2008) *Blogs, Wikis, Podcasts and Other Powerful Web Tools for Classrooms*. Thousand Oaks, CA: Corwin Press.

Sashek, J. (2004) Exerlearning: movement, fitness, dance, and learning. Unpublished Report. Sunnyvale, CA: RedOctane.

Smith, P., Rudd, P. and Coghlan, M. (2008) *Harnessing Technology: Schools Survey 2008*. Coventry: British Educational Communications and Technology Agency.

Tan B., Aziz, A.R., Chua, K. and The, K.C. (2001) Aerobic demands of the dance simulation game, *International Journal of Sports Medicine*, 23(2), pp. 125–129.

Unnithan, V.B., Houser, W. and Fernhall, B. (2006) Evaluation of the energy cost of playing a dance simulation video game in overweight and non-overweight children and adolescents, *International Journal of Sports Medicine*, 27(10), pp. 804–809.

Wood, J. (2005) *Body and Mind: A Report on the Use of ICT in Physical Education*. Coventry: British Educational Communications and Technology Agency.

Teaching for Examination

Jon Spence

This chapter provides teachers of physical education with some background, advice and areas for consideration when teaching for examinations in the subject. The chapter focuses on the approaches used to enhance teaching and learning as the content of the examination syllabus as this will vary from country to country and depending on the level.

I hear and I forget. I see and I remember. I do and I understand.

(Attributed to Confucius)

Learning is more than a test of memory and pupils need to be taught to understand and apply rather than to just recall. The above 'quote' from Confucius clearly exemplifies the philosophy behind this chapter and the secret to ensuring students achieve their full potential when sitting examinations in physical education.

Chapter 14 in this book identifies the plethora of different perspectives of learning and their application. All teachers need to consider how their pupils learn and what approaches are most appropriate to the topic being taught and the group who are to learn. Achieving an appropriate mix of teaching and learning approaches will help pupils succeed in physical education exams. Learning for examinations in physical education must focus on the underpinning *knowledge* and *understanding* of the concepts in a practical situation. Knowledge without understanding will not allow the pupil to achieve at the highest levels.

Conceptions of Learning

Key to this chapter is what in philosophical terms is the distinction between the *learning how* and the *learning that*. The philosopher Gilbert Ryle identified the difference between the *'that'* and the *'how'* suggesting that we can acquire factual knowledge by hearing or reading whereas we learn how to do something through doing it (Ryle, 1949). Learning *'the how'* and *'the that'* are both important in physical education and teaching needs to cater for both. Pupils need to develop knowledge and also to develop the cognitive skills to construct, reconstruct and evaluate what they know and what they do if they are to truly understand. It is therefore important that pupils are not just introduced to facts, but that they are also given the opportunity to apply and develop their knowledge and their cognitive skills if they are to succeed in the subject.

As physical educationalists we have always provided pupils with the opportunity to learn how to do things in the practical elements of the subject, however as Wagner (2002) identifies, we must allow learners to learn cognitive skills through doing. He suggests that facts are useless (if not meaningless) if one does not know what to do with them. In other words, if pupils do not have the opportunity to apply their knowledge through active learning approaches, be they practical sporting activities or cognitive learning activities, their knowledge is of little use as they only learn that rather than how.

> ### Reflection
>
> Consider the theoretical content of your teaching. Is the knowledge of the concept of use without knowing how to apply it?
>
> For example, you may know the effects of exercise on the body, but if you are unable to use that knowledge to improve performance then what is the point of knowing it!

Why Is Teaching for Examinations in Physical Education Different?

It's not! Good teaching is the same in all subjects. It does not matter whether it is to be formally examined or not. Good teaching will ensure that ALL pupils' needs are catered for and that learning goes beyond knowledge and skill. The teacher needs to provide the pupil with the theoretical knowledge and detailed understanding which allows them to apply the theoretical concepts to a range of different practical contexts.

Seven principles of good teaching (adapted from Chickering and Gamson, 1987)

Encourages interaction
A good teacher is able to provide activities and environments where the learner feels comfortable and is given the opportunity to interact with the topic and the teacher.

Develops reciprocity and co-operation among learners
A good teacher is able to provide a learning environment which involves pupils learning and working together.

Encourages active learning
A good teacher involves pupils in higher order thinking.

Gives prompt feedback
A good teacher give immediate and constructive feedback which helps pupils understand what they have done well and how they can improve.

Emphasizes time on task
A good teacher recognizes the importance of pupil involvement and plans for and provides appropriate time on learning activities to ensure full understanding.

Communicates high expectations
A good teacher encourages pupils to achieve their full potential and communicates their belief in the pupils through setting high expectations in terms of achievement and behaviour.

Respects diverse talents and ways of learning
A good teacher is aware of the individual differences of pupils and is able to cater for the differing needs and preferred learning styles of those being taught.

These principles should be remembered when considering the content of this chapter.

The Concept

Traditionally teachers of physical education have been trained to teach the practical aspects of the subject with much less attention paid to the teaching of theoretical concepts and classroom/examination based teaching. With an expansion in the formal examination of pupils' knowledge and skills across the world, the role of, and the demands placed on the physical education teacher have changed and evidence from Initial Teacher Training providers across England, Australia and other European countries would suggest that in many cases the training has not evolved accordingly. This chapter aims to identify how the physical education teacher can use their skills to develop appropriate pedagogical approaches to ensure that their pupils achieve their full potential in the classroom and the examined aspects of the subject. The need to teach the theoretical aspects of the subject has implications for Initial Teacher Training, CPD and the individual teacher.

The essentials for teaching pupils to achieve well in examinations in physical education are no different to those in any other subject. A compelling and memorable learning experience will help develop pupils understanding and will motivate them for future involvement in physical activity and study in the area. The key is to use approaches which enable pupils to gain the required depth of knowledge and a practical understanding of how the theoretical concepts can be applied. A variety of teaching approaches need to be used to meet the individual needs of pupils and also to suit the subject area within physical education. The teacher needs to develop an in depth understanding of the examination specification/syllabus and detailed knowledge/understanding of the theoretical aspects to be taught. This will help them to develop innovative approaches to teaching and the confidence to take risks in the teaching approaches they adopt.

Central to the successful teaching of the theoretical aspects of the subject is an understanding of the learning needs of those to be taught. The majority of pupils who opt to study physical education and to be examined in the subject are practical by nature and as such are aesthetic learners. The subject is underpinned by the practical elements of the course and therefore these aspects must remain central to any pedagogical debate and decisions. Teaching of theoretical concepts should be, as far as practicably possible, practical and applied. Learning should focus on the development of both knowledge and understanding and should be measured in the same way. Knowledge without understanding will not enable pupils to gain the highest marks and will not hold them in good stead for future learning in the subject.

Active Learning Approaches

The importance of 'active learning' approaches has been highlighted by Bonwell and Eison (1991) and many government and educational policy developments are founded on the premise that active approaches to learning will develop understanding and not just superficial knowledge. Most important, to be actively involved, students must engage in such higher-order thinking tasks as analysis, synthesis and evaluation. Within this context, it is proposed that strategies promoting active learning be defined as instructional activities involving students in doing things and thinking about what they are doing (Bonwell and Eison, 1991). To the teacher of physical education active and practical approaches to learning are not unusual, however it is important to recognize that these should involve thinking as well as doing. The concept of developing understanding as well as knowledge has been adopted by many examining authorities and examining agencies nationally and internationally where exams demand pupils to apply knowledge to a wide range of practical situations and to explain the 'how' and the 'why' rather than the 'what', this encourages pupils to become analytical and reflective.

Reflection

Reflect on the extent to which your pupils develop knowledge and understanding.
Can your pupils answer factual questions such as:

- Name a particular bone
- What is Newton's first law?
- When were the Sydney Olympic Games?

If the answer is yes, then that is great, they have developed knowledge, but can they answer questions such as:

- How do Newton's Laws influence performance in the Javelin?
- Explain how a performer who has lost a game might be motivated to train harder and to perform better next time?

The second set of questions, those which are the 'how' and the 'why' and those which require explanation and links to the sporting context are those which we must focus on and which pupils will need to be able to answer if they are to perform well in exams. Examiners are looking for applied knowledge and understanding of how the theory can be applied to different sporting contexts, not just to test the ability to remember. Bloom's Taxonomy (Bloom et al., 1956) demonstrates the importance of the cognitive domain and the 'levels' of learning required to achieve well in examinations in physical education are clear in his analysis of the cognitive domain:

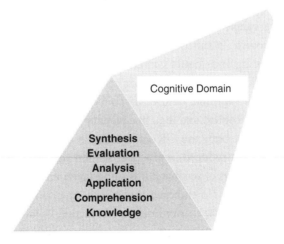

Figure 11.1 Bloom's taxonomy (adapted from Bloom et al., 1956).

Achievement of full understanding and ultimately improved achievement in examinations in physical education requires learning beyond knowledge and comprehension. Pupils need to apply, analyse, synthesize and evaluate if they are to truly learn.

The importance of a coherent, integrated and practical approach to teaching theoretical concepts through practical learning activities has been demonstrated in the following case study.

Case Study

A school in the South of England, whose pupils had consistently underperformed in formal physical education exams when compared to other schools and to other subjects in their school. The teaching team reviewed their teaching approaches and the range of learning activities and recognized that their pupils had developed good theoretical knowledge but underperformed in written exams.

The physical education staff reviewed the teaching approaches used across the two years of the course and identified where the theoretical concepts could be placed into practical learning environments. This change required careful planning and flexibility in timetabling to allow access to a theoretical and practical learning space during every lesson enabling concepts to be introduced in the classroom and then practical learning activities to be developed. Results improved markedly over the following two years and teachers felt much more comfortable using this combined approach providing contextual learning opportunities rather than a purely theoretical approach.

To what extent do your pupils develop understanding? Do they know the theory? Can they apply the theory to practical examples?

This book is not advocating that all theoretical aspects of the physical education curriculum should be taught through the practical, more that the pupils should learn to apply the theory to a range of practical concepts. Introducing applied/active learning activities needs to be logical, planned and real, not contrived. Learning activities should contribute to understanding and should cement learning if they are to be of value. When asked to recount their most memorable lessons, pupils in the UK, the Netherlands and Australia all described lessons where theoretical concepts were introduced, then they were demonstrated in a practical context and then in a plenary session the learning was reinforced and tested. In fact pupils in both the UK and Australia described similar lessons where the topic of feedback was introduced, a practical session involving shooting a basketball blindfolded with different types of feedback was undertaken and then discussion about the activity took place. The pupils remembered the theory, experienced the impact and were able to discuss and explain how the theory influenced practice. Details of the feedback lesson are included below to demonstrate the structure of a memorable lesson which developed both knowledge and understanding and which enabled pupils to apply their knowledge to a range of sporting contexts.

> **Exemplar Active Learning Lesson**
>
> ## Theoretical introduction (classroom-based)
> What is feedback?
> Types of feedback
>
> - Positive or negative?
> - Terminal or concurrent
>
> Forms of feedback
>
> - Verbal or visual or kinaesthetic?
> - Knowledge of results or knowledge of performance?
>
> ## Practical application (sports hall-based)
> ## Impact of feedback
> A pupil shoots a basketball from the free throw line 5 times counting 2 points for scoring and 1 for hitting the ring:
>
> - Attempt 1 – no feedback
> - Attempt 2 – verbal feedback about the result after each shot, that is, missed or scored
> - Attempt 3 – verbal feedback about the outcome, that is, missed short left etc.
> - Attempt 4 – as in 3 but shooter is manipulated into position each time before shooting to ensure they know exactly where the basket is.

This chapter does not deal with the theoretical aspects surrounding learning. Chapter 14 covers four theoretical perspectives, namely, behaviourist, cognitivist, situated learning and the organic viewpoint categorized by Greeno et al. (1996) and Davis et al. (2008). The approaches advocated in this chapter would appear to fit most closely with simple definitions of situational learning as identified by Lave and Wenger (1991), that is, that situated learning is learning that takes place in the same context in which it is applied. Lave and Wenger (1991) argue that learning should not be viewed as simply the transmission of abstract and decontextualized knowledge from one individual to another, but a social process whereby knowledge is co-constructed; they suggest that such learning is situated in a specific context and embedded within a particular social and physical environment. The specific nature of learning for a subject or particular activity would make the term 'contextual learning' most appropriate in the discussions in this chapter.

Work with students studying for qualifications in physical education across London has shown that many of the students studying for examinations in physical education are doing so because they enjoy and excel in the practical aspects of the subject. Examinations in physical education across the world assess not only the practical performance but also require assessment of theoretical knowledge. Interestingly the examination of theoretical aspects of the subject has remained true to the practical nature of the subject, requiring contextual and applied knowledge and understanding rather than abstract knowledge. Pupils who have good theoretical knowledge will not necessarily perform to their best in examinations in physical education as they are unable to adapt their knowledge. Contextual learning which has enabled the pupil to develop knowledge of a theoretical concept, to see the theory applied to a practical situation and then provides the opportunity to transfer this understanding to a range of other contexts will better prepare pupils to answer questions fully in an examination and to show examiners that they have the depth of knowledge and understanding required to achieve the highest grades.

Reflection

In your teaching, how can you help pupils to develop their contextual knowledge and their ability to apply their knowledge to a range of different sporting contexts even if they know very little about the particular sport? For example, how can you teach a pupil who is a weak swimmer to apply biomechanical principles to the Breast Stroke kick?

In many schools, models of Sport Education (Siedentop, 1994) and Teaching Games for Understanding (Thorpe et al., 1986) are used to improve learning in physical education and building on these concepts will enable pupils to achieve the higher grades in the examined aspects of the subject. Evidence from Examination board reports and OfSTED inspection reports and observation of teachers in a range of different schools would suggest that due to a lack of training or possibly a lack of confidence, physical education teachers appear to revert back to didactic, classroom-based approaches to teaching when covering theoretical concepts and preparing pupils for examinations. In schools who perform well in terms of examination results there is clear evidence that pupils learn through active approaches and in many of these schools, examination classes are not just timetabled in the classroom. Lessons take place in the classroom and in a practical facility to allow theory to be applied. In a large college in England where pupils perform well above the national average, every physical education lesson is timetabled in a classroom and with a practical facility. In a typical 1-hour lesson at the college, the class will spend just 20 minutes in the classroom and may move between the practical facility and the classroom several times in the lesson.

Reflection

What practical learning activities do you use in your teaching? Do you use these activities to maximize learning? Can pupils see a clear relationship between the theory and the practical learning episode?

In order to maximize learning and understanding, it is important to review the curriculum and the examination requirements to identify active and contextual learning opportunities. Active/contextual learning activities require careful planning if the opportunity is to be maximized. The learning activities need to be memorable and appropriate if they are to help pupils to develop a greater understanding and if they are to be able to apply practical examples to theoretical concepts. As a team, a physical education department need to identify the theoretical concepts which can be applied and they need to devise a series of practical learning activities which work together to allow a range of theories to be related and a synoptic knowledge to be developed and to ensure fully rounded and physically educated pupils.

Some examples of learning activities which can be used to ensure understanding of specific theoretical concepts are included below. This list is not prescriptive and the teacher needs to develop activities to suit the individual needs of their own pupils.

Examples of Learning Activities

Figure 11.2 gives examples of learning activities used in schools to develop theoretical knowledge and understanding and utilizing practical learning approaches.

Theoretical concept	Learning activity
Circulatory systems	System modelling: • Organize pupils into groups to perform the different components, i.e. breathing, heart, lungs, oxygen transportation, muscles etc. • Demonstrate the process of taking in oxygen, transferring it into the lungs, transferring into the blood and then pumping the oxygenated blood via the heart to the muscles. • Using coloured balls to represent oxygenated and deoxygenated blood helps pupils understand the process
Attribution theory	Sporting competition/match • Organize a sporting competition/match amongst the pupils. • Following the competition pupils will then need to identify reasons for the outcomes. For example, played well, luck, referee decisions, opposition better etc. • The discussions about the results can then be applied to Weiner's theory of attribution (Weiner, 1980, 1992). • Theories of motivation can then be used to demonstrate how performance can be improved through the application of theories of motivation.

Figure 11.2 Continued.

Skill acquisition: stages of learning	Select a skill which pupils cannot perform (e.g. juggling)
	Take them through the different stages of learning to help them acquire the skill:
	• Cognitive stage
	Demonstrate the skill so they can form a mental picture of what needs to be done. Explain how the skill is performed
	• Associative stage
	Give pupils time to practice, give feedback and demonstrate again as appropriate.
Introduction of other learning/teaching theories	• Autonomous stage
	Can the pupils achieve the autonomous stage in the skill? How do they know if they have?
	To help pupils learn the skill and understand other theories the teacher can introduce parts methods of information presentation, task simplification (use of balloons, beanbags etc.), different types of feedback, practice conditions etc. This could take place over a number of weeks/lessons using the initial skill as a mechanism to demonstrate the different theories/approaches to teaching and learning in the physical domain.
Moment of inertia	Speed of rotation
	• Using trampolining or gymnastics, video a pupil from different angles jumping and rotating in different positions – Fully extended, tucked arms out etc.
	• Pupils can then use the video to identify speeds of rotation in different positions
	• There are a range of other practical activities which involve rotation and which pupils can experiment to gain further understanding of body position and the position of the centre of gravity on rotation
Attention/concentration/ social facilitation	Fine motor skill performance
	• Ask pupils to perform a fine motor skill under different conditions such as alone, in competition, in front of an audience, with other distractions etc.
	• Performance in the different conditions can then be analysed by outcome and in terms of the performer's feelings whilst performing.
	• Various theories/concepts can be introduced/linked to the activity focusing on the psychological factors impacting on performance and how to improve performance.
Performance analysis	Performer commentary
	• Many examinations in physical education across the world require pupils to be able to analyse performance. Pupils will watch sport and listen to the commentary regularly but this often is descriptive rather than analytical.
	• Pupils can be asked to include a commentary on a live or recorded performance.
	• Pupils can be given an aide memoir which highlights areas to comment on. They should be encouraged to comment on technical aspects of the performance – what is good and why, what is less good and how can it be improved.
	• Recording the commentary provides an excellent teaching resource which can be used to discuss analytical skills as well as to practice for examinations.

Figure 11.2 Examples of learning activities.

Preparing for Examinations

Performing well in examinations is more than just about knowing and understanding the subject. As in sport, if you practice you get better, you can't expect to perform well if you don't work hard at your technique and if you don't know the rules you are unlikely to succeed. Teaching pupils to perform well in the examination aspects of physical education requires teachers to provide pupils with the factual information, help them to develop the understanding which enables them to apply theory to practice and to help them to understand what examiners are asking and what they are looking for in an answer. Many of the principles hold for all examinations, others relate specifically to physical education examinations.

Practical Guidance for Examination Preparation

There are a number of key principles that teachers need to ensure pupils are aware of and to which they need to adhere when they are sitting examinations, including:

Read and follow the instructions carefully (pupils should have practiced so know what they should do, but reading helps reduce stress and ensures mistakes are not made).
   Many pupils answer more questions than required; the extras generally will not be marked.

Plan time appropriately (work out how many minutes can be allocated to each mark).
   The later marks in a question are often harder to gain than the early ones in the next.

Answer the question (look carefully at the words used, describe, exemplify, illustrate, justify etc. all examination terms should be familiar to pupils if they are to do well).
   Many pupils write what they know, not what the question asks! The marking criteria will identify what points need to be made and only the equivalent answers will be accepted.

Always write in sentences unless the question asks for a list.
   Many examination systems give marks for the way the answer is written and marks will be lost for poor spelling and grammar.

Plan your answers and hand the plans in.
   Examiners will give credit for what's in the plan.

Look at the marks awarded (the marks available will generally identify how many different points a pupil needs to make).
   Often a mark will be available for each point and a further mark for a sporting example.

Always exemplify with a sporting example (even when examples are not asked for, you should try to include one. Remember, physical education is an 'applied science').
   Don't always use the same sport in your examples as examiners will think you only know about one and lack depth of knowledge.

Underline/highlight key points.
   Make the job of the marker easy by underlining or using subheadings. This will help them see that you have included the key points required to be awarded the marks.

Working with a large range of pupils and preparing them for examinations in the subject has demonstrated the importance of developing detailed understanding of theoretical concepts and equally important, preparing them for the examination. Practice of examination technique will enable pupils to go into the examination with confidence. Whether the examination is written or practical, preparation is key. As a teacher you must understand what the examiner is looking for and you must understand how the examinations are marked. Often the best way to gain an insight into the examination requirements is to work as a marker. Examining bodies are often looking for teachers to work as markers, by doing this you will be trained and you will begin to understand what you need to do to prepare your pupils better for their examinations.

Reflection

Consider the examinations you are preparing your pupils for, look back at past questions and make a list of the key words which occur in the questions, for example, illustrate, explain etc.
Write an explanation for each of the recurring terms.

Conclusion

This chapter has provided some ideas to help better prepare your pupils for examinations in physical education. The intention was to stimulate thought about how to make teaching more active/contextual and how to maximize learning and ultimately to improve examination performance. The teacher needs to review the curriculum and understand the learners' requirements to identify appropriate active learning activities that can be used.

Learning More

Further sources are available to help you provide a high quality learning experience for your pupils. You should utilize the texts provided by the specific examining authority and familiarize yourself with the syllabus/specification in detail. Sources to assist in the planning and implementation of Sport Education are available (e.g. Hastie and Kinchin, 2004; Siedentop, Hastie and van der Mars, 2004). Some texts have been written for specific use of co-operative learning in physical education (Grineski, 1996). Some TGfU sources are available for those interested in putting this instructional approach into practice (e.g. Griffin, et al., 1997; Mitchell et al., 2003).

References

Bloom, B.S., Englehart, M.D., Furst, E.J., Hill, W.H. and Krathwohl, D.R. (1956) *Taxonomy of Educational Objectives. Handbook 1: Cognitive Domain.* New York: Longmans, Green.

Bonwell, C.C. and Eison, J. (1991) *Active Learning: Creating Excitement in the Classroom AEHE-ERIC Higher Education Report No.1.* Washington, DC: Jossey-Bass.

Chickering A.W. and Gamson Z.F. (1987) Seven principles for good practice in undergraduate education, *American Association of Higher Education Bulletin*, pp. 3–7.

Davis, B., Sumara, D. and Luce-Kapler, R. (2008) *Engaging Minds: Changing Teaching in Complex Times.* Second edition. New York: Routledge.

Griffin, L.L., Mitchell, S.A. and Oslin, J.L. (1997) *Teaching Sport Concepts and Skills: A Tactical Games Approach.* Champaign, IL, Human Kinetics.

Grineski, S. (1996) *Cooperative Learning in Physical Education.* Champaign, IL: Human Kinetics.

Greeno, J.G., Collins, A.M. and Resnick, L.B. (1996) Cognition and learning (pp. 15–46). In D.C. Berliner and R.C. Calfee (eds), *Handbook of Educational Psychology.* New York: Simon and Schuster/Macmillan.

Hastie, P. and Kinchin, G.D. (2004). Design a season of sport education, *British Journal of Teaching Physical Education*, 35(1), pp. 14–18.

Lave, J. and Wenger, E. (1991) *Situated Learning. Legitimate Peripheral Participation*, Cambridge: Cambridge University Press.

Mitchell, S.A., Oslin, J.L., and Griffin, L.L. (2003) *Sport Foundations for Elementary Physical Education: A Tactical Games Approach.* Champaign, IL: Human Kinetics.

Ryle, G. (1949) *The Concept of Mind.* London: Hutchinson.

Siedentop, D. (1994) The sport education model (pp. 3–16). In D. Siedentop (ed.), *Sport Education: Quality PE through Positive Sport Experiences.* Champaign, IL: Human Kinetics.

Siedentop, D., Hastie, P.A. and van der Mars, H. (2004) *Complete Guide to Sport Education.* Champaign, IL: Human Kinetics.

Thorpe, R., Bunker, D. and Almond, L. (eds) (1986) *Rethinking Games Teaching.* Loughborough: University of Technology, Loughborough.

Wagner, R.H. (2002) Knowing, learning and teaching. Unpublished essay http://web.austin.utexas.edu/hw/papers/klt.pdf

12 Working with Partners

Lesley Phillpots

This chapter investigates the increasing demands placed upon physical education teachers to work with a range of partners beyond the school context. These changes have been driven by political demands to raise academic standards in schools and to improve the quality of teaching and learning for all pupils. As a physical education teacher you will be expected to work with a range of partners outside the school environment in order to provide high quality physical education and school sport (PESS) for your pupils and your local community. This chapter explains the rationale underpinning the concept of working in partnership and evaluates the benefits and challenges that this poses for the physical education teacher.

In the UK, partnership working has become the organizational strategy most strongly espoused as a means of achieving policy goals within education. The requirement for schools to work in partnership with external agencies has not been confined to the UK; indeed this approach reflects developments worldwide. In Australia, the Victoria Government's Report

(2000) on '*Public Education*' provided strong research evidence that pupil learning could be measurably strengthened by a genuine commitment to partnership working. In the case of physical education, Marshall and Hardman reported that municipal, regional, county and national level partnership networks existed in 70 per cent of the countries surveyed world-wide. Links between school physical education departments and sports organizations occurred on a regular basis, with many countries recording obligatory partnerships between physical education departments and community physical activity settings (Marshall and Hardman, 2000). Physical education teachers now operate in school environments where there is an expectation that they will engage with, and also take the lead in, managing partnerships to benefit the children they teach. The landscape for partnership working has never been more pronounced.

If physical education teachers are to be effective in ensuring that partnerships work, it is incumbent upon them to engage with, and seek to understand, the complexities and challenges that this presents. This chapter explores the general principles underpinning the concept of 'partnership' and 'partnership working' and provides practitioners and students with an insight into the roles of the key agencies with whom they are likely to engage. Practical examples of good practice in partnership working are provided through four UK case studies which illustrate how these arrangements in have enhanced standards of learning and performance in physical education.

Partnership Working and Physical Education

Academic literature contains considerable discussion of the meaning and definition of partnership. Whilst it is acknowledged that there is a lack of coherence in the definition of what actually constitutes partnership, there is a general consensus that it involves an agreement between two or more parties that have consented to work together in the pursuit of common goals. A useful definition is provided by the UK Audit Commission (1998) who highlight the importance of

> joint working arrangements where parties who are otherwise independent bodies agree to co-operate to achieve common goals, create a new organisational structure or process to achieve these goals, who plan and implement a joint programme and share relevant information, tasks and rewards. (p. 32)

In the UK, the election of New Labour in 1997 led to a strategic focus upon partnership working as a key mechanism for effective and efficient public service delivery. For schools, this meant that they now had a 'duty of partnership' to work with a range of agencies for the benefit of all their pupils. Sue Campbell (in her position as Chief Executive of the Youth Sport Trust) acknowledged the challenges that this posed for physical education, but urged all partners involved in the delivery of PESS to work together in the interests of young people, whilst retaining their individual integrity (PEA/UK, 1997). This new emphasis upon partnership working coincided with the introduction of the *Physical Education, School Sport and Club Links* (PESSCL) strategy (DfES/DCMS, 2002). It was a new infrastructure aimed at transforming PESS in England and was predominantly based upon a number of key partnerships between government departments, schools, Local Education Authorities and sports agencies. The PESSCL strategy was a conglomeration of initiatives and work strands combined into a single overarching strategy. Schools had a pivotal role to play in enhancing the take-up of sporting opportunities for young people by pooling and linking their resources in collaborative arrangements with local and regional sport and community providers.

A Partnership Infrastructure for PESS

The National Strategy for PESS was delivered through an infrastructure of partnership arrangements that focused upon delivery of a government public service agreement (PSA) target to increase the percentage of school children in England engaged in a minimum of two hours each week on high quality PESS within and beyond the curriculum (DfES, DCMS, 2003). The UK Government's investment was monitored closely through a PSA target which required all partner organizations to deliver high quality and efficient services (Cabinet Office, 1999, p. 1). PSAs were a tool used by government to ensure that all partners were responsible for improved priority setting and the delivery of performance targets (James, 2004). The allocation of a PSA target for physical education accelerated the combined work of all the partners engaged in the delivery of PESSCL strategy and placed accountability on all the agencies involved (Penney and Houlihan, 2001).

The PESSCL Strategy

The national strategy was delivered through nine interlinked work strands which are described below:

1. Sports Colleges   Sports colleges receive government and private funding to raise standards of achievement in physical education and sport thus securing whole school improvement. They act as regional focal points for promoting excellence in physical education and community sport, extending links between families of schools, sports bodies and communities, sharing resources and developing and spreading good practice. Sports colleges were expected to promote a visible sports ethos throughout the school and within their local community.

2. School Sport Partnerships

School Sport Partnerships operate as families of schools and receive additional funding from government to enhance sports opportunities for all. These partnerships include all maintained schools in England and are typically clustered around a specialist sports college. They are managed by a full-time partnership development manager whose role is to develop and manage the partnership. Secondary school partners appoint a school sport co-ordinator (an existing teacher from the physical education department) who is released from the timetable to work with a cluster of primary schools to develop after school activities and links with local community and sports clubs.

3. School/club links

This work strand strengthens links between schools and local sports clubs and increase the number of children who are members of accredited sports clubs. The programme is delivered through partnership arrangements between schools and governing bodies of sport. The target is to increase the percentage of 5- to 16-year-olds from School Sport Partnership schools who are members of, or participate in, governing body or accredited sports clubs.

4. Gifted and Talented

The principle aim is to improve the identification of, support and provision for gifted and talented pupils in PESS. Talent support programmes are delivered through School Sport Partnerships to help talented young people. Physical education teachers work with a range of partners to support pupils within the curriculum and in their lifestyle management and performance planning.

5. Step Into Sport

A framework of co-ordinated opportunities at a local level to enable young people to begin and sustain involvement in leadership and volunteering through sport. Physical education teachers work with a range of partners so their pupils can experience sports leadership, gain leadership qualifications, help children in primary schools organize festivals of sport, and take up sports volunteering placements in their communities.

6. Sporting Playgrounds

Focuses upon tackling inactivity, boredom and poor behaviour by improving playtimes in primary schools. Sponsored by Nike and based upon playground zones, the model aims to increase physical activity levels and improve behaviour in schools.

7. Swimming

To ensure children are able to swim unaided over a distance of at least 25 metres, schools and local authorities strengthen partnerships between public, private and voluntary sectors and established clear swimming strategies in consultation with parents and the wider community.

8. QCA PE and School Sport Investigation

The QCA (a public body sponsored by the UK Government) worked with primary, secondary, special schools and partnerships across England to develop ways of improving the quality of PESS and to explore the difference that high quality PESS made to young people and their schools.

On completion of the project it was reported that high quality PESS had made schools happier, healthier and more successful and pupils had improved self-esteem and had achieved higher standards.

9. Professional development

In order to ensure high-quality PESS, physical education teachers are supported by a range of in-service modules that provide the tools and expertise needed to inspire and engage children and young people.

Reflection

The PESSCL strategy served a complex range of education, sport and community agendas through a network of partnership arrangements that involved diverse organizations working to collective outcomes. It placed an explicit requirement upon Physical Education teachers to forge links with sport agencies outside the school context. Consider the three school contexts below and to make a list of the partners and sport agencies with which Physical Education teachers in each of these schools may engage.

- Secondary schools (11–18 years)
- Primary schools (4–11 years)
- Special schools

Specialist sports colleges, school sports partnerships (SSPs) and national governing bodies were key agencies involved in delivering the PSA target for PESS. They were required to work in partnership to provide a seamless link between high quality physical education and high quality community sport. Their key roles and responsibilities are outlined in more detail below.

Specialist Sports Colleges

The UK's 1997 Labour government's vision for physical education and sport was predominantly realized though the work of Specialist Sports Colleges. As a condition of their funding arrangements with government, sports colleges were required to raise sporting and academic standards in schools and maintain an active role in establishing and driving partnerships between schools, the private sector and the wider community (Evans et al., 2002; DfES, 2003). The expectation was that specialist schools were outward looking in seeking innovative and collaborative practices in order to improve attainment and achievement within their own school and that of their partner schools. This approach to partnership working was a new challenge for schools that were more used to working in a competitive, rather than co-operative local education market. Sports colleges were required to allocate a proportion of their budget to support the work of SSPs by acting as regional hubs of excellence in physical education and community sport (Penney and Houlihan, 2001). This new educational milieu for schools was based upon government demands for increased partnership collaboration. It meant that a physical education teacher's role now involved working with local businesses and community groups, sports clubs, governing bodies and sports development units in order to provide sustainable sporting opportunities which promoted both participation and achievement in physical education and community sport (DfEE, 2000). Based within a Specialist Sports College, Directors of Sport (or Specialism) 'project managed' these new strategic partnerships ensuring that PESS contributed to whole-school development and improvement.

Reflection

The extract below is from an interview with a Director of Sport at a large sports college in Central England. It provides an insight into the responsibilities placed upon secondary schools and Physical Education staff to work in partnership with sports agencies and partners in the community.

> Our teachers are coming up with more new and innovative ideas that stretch the boundaries of learning and opportunity further than ever before. As a Director of Specialism you have to plan your priorities and balance needs against available funding. It is important that the Physical Education Department reaches beyond the school into the wider community in order to create opportunities for local people. I also need to make sure my own Physical Education department's priorities are not overlooked. Often this means employing extra staff and creates an extra tier of management. When we first became a sports college, several members of staff were given additional responsibility points to allow them to carry out specific projects associated with the specialism, such as continuing professional development, liaising with local sports clubs and providing leadership courses in sport. It's not enough though to simply provide for those students who already like sport, if a particular activity is popular and there is no one on the staff with the necessary expertise, then either staff training must be arranged or outside professionals brought in. At a sports college such as ours, this might include street dance, judo, yoga, tri-golf or cheerleading. My role increasingly involves me networking with a range of partners outside school in order to achieve our targets and objectives.

Whilst schools have offered a broader range of sports activities beyond the curriculum context, the PESSCL strategy has had a limited impact upon the quality of the Physical Education curriculum in schools. Reflect upon this statement and consider the challenges that Physical Education teachers may encounter in balancing the demands of delivering the Physical Education curriculum and their community sport responsibilities.

School Sport Partnerships

School Sport Partnerships (SSPs) represented a significant element of the infrastructure of the PESSCL strategy based upon local networks of schools that typically included a specialist sports college, approximately 8 secondary schools and 45 primary schools clustered around them (DfES, 2003). The work of specialist sports colleges and SSPs were intended to be mutually supportive with the SSPs key remit to ensure the delivery of the PSA target for PESS. By forging meaningful relationships with community providers, the SSP was responsible for ensuring all young people continued to play sport in a community environment. A typical SSP model and its core personnel are provided below.

Core partnership roles

Partnership Development Manager (PDM)

A full time strategic management position, usually based at a sports college, a PDM is responsible for the management and development of the partnership. Their role is to link with other physical education and sport organizations within, between and beyond schools.

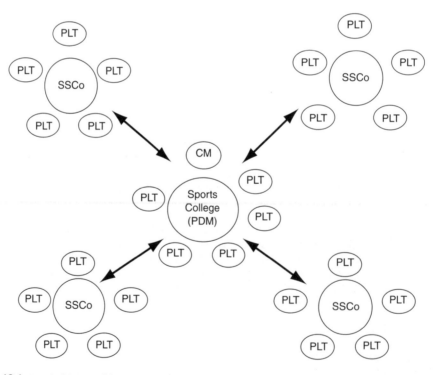

Figure 12.1 A typical SSP model.

School Sport Co-ordinator (SSCo)

An existing secondary school teacher released from teaching for two days per week, an SSCo divides time between the secondary school and cluster primary schools to co-ordinate and develop school sport opportunities and community sport pathways.

Primary Link Teacher (PLT)

A primary or special school teacher released from teaching for 12 days per year, a PLT advocates high quality physical education, co-ordinates and supports school sport opportunities.

Competition Manager (CM)

This is a full time position responsible for the modernization of the local competition landscape by strategically developing opportunities to increase the number of young people taking part in inter-school competition.

The main responsibilities shared by all these core partnership roles included strategic leadership and management, delivery and access to high quality physical education and sport for all young people in school and community contexts and the provision of coaching, leading and volunteering opportunities. The outcomes represented a mixture of education, sport and community objectives and underlined the challenges for all the partners involved in working together to deliver these objectives.

Reflection

The extract below is from an interview with a PDM who has been working at a sports college for over five years. It provides an insight into the responsibilities placed upon PDMs to develop and managing partnerships within, between and beyond schools.

> As a Partnership Development Manager I lead and manage the work of the partnership. I do this by, setting clear targets whilst also developing and nurturing relationships with key partners such as local schools and local sports clubs. To achieve the outcomes for my SSP, I have to negotiate with head teachers, directors of specialism, local education authorities, local authority sports development units, the Youth Sport Trust, County Sport Partnerships, Sport England and the Big Lottery Fund. In order to do this I have received training support from the Youth Sport Trust to help me achieve my objectives and to work more effectively with other partners. I also have to ensure that there are opportunities for talented young school children to access high quality performance opportunities as part of a wider strategic, sustainable coaching development remit. This is a challenging array of education, sport and community partners for a single PDM to deal with.

PDMs need the skills to network and to lead and manage staff. These skills have been highlighted as the ability to:

- create a positive, inclusive and responsive climate to develop your vision;
- manage individuals and teams effectively;
- provide effective professional development for your staff; and
- review the performance of your staff and yourself.

Analyse your own skill set and consider whether this role might be appeal to you at some time in your future career.

The National Governing Bodies (NGBs) of Sport

The election of the UK Labour Government in 1997 led to a fundamental change in its funding relationship with NGBs. Their perceived overdependence on public funds led to the introduction of *Whole Sport Plans* in 2003 which provided new lines of accountability through which they were managed and controlled. For NGBs, the acquisition of government funding was contingent upon their willingness to adhere to new contractual funding conditions which contained explicit agreements to work with schools to support the delivery of the government's PESSCL strategy (Garrett, 2004). The PSA target placed an explicit demand on both schools and NGBs to work in partnership. This was a marked departure from previous practices where physical education teachers had been reluctance to allow sports coaches to work in schools. Ideological arguments surrounding the nature of physical education and sport stifled any attempts by governing bodies to make formal linkages and partnerships with schools. Philosophical arguments about the nature of physical education and sport have been well documented and the debates are still ongoing (see, for example, Penney and Evans, 1997; Evans and Penney, 1998; Kirk and Gorely, 2000; Kay, 2003). The introduction of the PESSCL strategy meant that schools and NGBs had to work in partnership to deliver a joint PSA target. Government funding became contingent upon the willingness of schools and NGBs to adhere to these new contractual funding conditions and to support the delivery of the government's policy outcomes for PESS.

Reflection

The extract below is from an interview conducted with a Chief Executive of a major governing body for sport. It provides an account of the responsibilities placed upon them by the PESSCL strategy to work in partnership with schools. Reflect upon its content, and consider as a teacher of Physical Education, your own attitude towards the involvement of governing bodies of sport in the delivery of PESS.

> For many years we had been struggling to work with schools that were either reluctant or did not have the time or funding to work with us on a systematic basis. The relationship we had with schools was ad hoc. The creation of this new infrastructure for Physical Education and sport in England meant that both NGBs and schools had to make formal agreements to work together. From an NGB's perspective, the creation of School Sport Partnerships and the appointment of PDMs made a significant difference to our access to young people and schools in particular. As a result, PDMs were on the top of our hit list, the network of PDMs and sport colleges gave us something new we could target. All of a sudden we could dramatically increase our reach into schools. I think that was solely down to the new network of school sport partnerships and PDMs and the efforts of Physical Education teachers who were now willing to work in partnership with us. It has made a remarkable difference to the amount of children that are now playing our sport both in schools and in our clubs.

Innovative Approaches to Working in Partnership

In order to provide detailed evidence of the benefits of the PESSCL strategy and the benefits of working through partnership arrangements, the QCA was asked by the Government to provide evidence of how schools were making improvements to the quality of PESS for all pupils. A key task was to exemplify good practice and to illustrate the impact that these new partnership arrangements had made in raising pupils' attainment in physical education and improving standards of performance in school sport.

The four case studies included in this chapter have been provided by the QCA. They are examples of innovative approaches to teaching, learning and assessment that emerged as a direct consequence of new partnership arrangements in PESS. They illustrate the changing demands placed upon physical education teachers to work with a network of external agencies and have been selected because they could be operationalized and implemented across a range of school settings worldwide.

Case Study 1

The key objective of this partnership initiative was to increase the percentage of pupils taking part in out-of-hours school sport. The sports college had already worked hard to establish an extensive programme of out-of-hours school sport with its sporting partners that included a nationally recognized athletics club, a Premiership football team, a national squad velodrome training facility and a local golf and country club. The sports college management group implemented a new strategy for all out-of-hours sport provision in which college staff were invited to apply for funded posts as out-of-hours learning co-coordinators. Staff were required to hold a relevant coaching qualification and expected to implement and manage sport development plans. The co-ordinators met twice a term as the 'out-of-hours sports management group' to agree outcomes and to consider how to make further progress with all the partners involved. The wide range of provision helped to ensure that activities were offered at a range of times, so that pupils were more likely to be able to attend. This reduced the barriers to participation such as transport difficulties, home commitments and part-time jobs for older pupils and resulted in more opportunities for all pupils to enhance their performance and learn new skills in a range of sports activities.

Case Study 2

This strategic partnership consisted of a group of schools brought together under the leadership of the Local Education Authority (LEA). The aim of this initiative was to increase pupils' activity levels, improve their progress in physical education generally and improve attitudes to learning through a particular focus on dance. The partnership had LEA support, used college students and coaches from the local community, made links with a disco dancing club and ran keep-fit clubs for both parents and children. As a result of the programme, the confidence and self-esteem of the pupils was assessed by the physical education staff as having increased considerably. The partnership arrangements meant that the target group of boys in particular had grown in confidence and their behaviour in and around school had generally improved.

Case Study 3

This partnership's agreed objectives were to increase the number of pupils involved in at least two hours' high quality physical education and sport each week and to tackle pupils' behaviour and attitudes to PESS at lunchtimes. To achieve these objectives, the physical education staff involved in the partnership decided to increase the amount of curriculum time they devoted to physical education each week. Partners included physical education teachers who linked with local Active Leisure and Healthy Schools co-ordinators, an LEA trainer who trained practitioners to help deliver through the Community Sports Leader Award (CSLA) and adult play workers who were all employed to increase the number of out-of-hours sports clubs on offer. All of the partners met regularly to share ideas and successes. As a result, more pupils in the school sport partnership received their entitlement to two hours of PESS a week. Behaviour improved across all the schools and there was a significant increase in the number of pupils involved in lunchtime activities and after-school sport. Attitudes to learning were also recorded as having improved significantly.

Case Study 4

The School Club Links initiative is a key strand of the PESSCL strategy that aims to provide seamless links from high quality school sport to high quality community sport in NGB-accredited sports clubs. School-club links were developed by physical education teachers with a local gymnastics club that had received *GymMark* accreditation enabling it to work with partner organizations within a school sport partnership. The head gymnastics coach worked in five schools in order to improve the confidence and knowledge and understanding of teachers responsible for delivering gymnastics in their schools. The objective of this initiative was to improve the quality of the delivery of the gymnastics curriculum within schools. The project was deemed as successful in its goal of improving the quality of teaching and learning in lessons as a direct consequence of the close partnership that had been forged between the teachers and the gymnastics coach. The benefits also extended to the children who showed an improvement in their body awareness which led to their increased enjoyment and willingness to learn in gymnastics.

The Benefits and Challenges of Working in Partnerships

Whilst these Case studies attest to the benefits of working in partnerships, it is important to be mindful of the particular challenges that are faced by physical education teachers in their efforts to co-ordinate the work of a number of partners. Donovan et al. (2006, p. 16) highlight the challenges and potential difficulties faced by teachers in delivering a national school sport strategy that attempts to reconcile 'the historical duality of physical education and sport, in partnership approaches'. Furthermore, they attest to the inherent difficulty in forging relationships between schools, sports clubs, teachers and coaches, who may have different education and sport agendas.

As the case studies reveal, partnership working is a potentially powerful tool in enhancing learning and performance opportunities for all pupils within physical education. The key ingredients for successful partnerships appear to be shared objectives; a clear framework of responsibilities and accountability and a high level of trust between the partners. Partnership working is undoubtedly a productive way of achieving more efficient and effective use of local resources. Nevertheless, partnership working between a range of agencies is often time consuming for teachers and therefore difficult to do well. As a consequence, the decision to get involved in working with other partners should only be undertaken when the goals and outcomes of the initiative outweigh the resources that they may consume. The PESSCL strategy undoubtedly brought schools closer to a range of public, private and voluntary agencies involved in the delivery of sport.

Conclusion

The complexities of partnership working present a challenge for physical education teachers who are at the hub of a range of education and sport policy initiatives (Green and Houlihan, 2005). Teachers are required to take the lead in managing partners from sport and community sectors that often operate on the basis of different professional norms, values and procedural systems (Hutt et al., 2000). The complex infrastructure of assorted sport agencies and policy initiatives that surround the work of schools means that physical education teachers require a skill set that allows them to manage physical education and sport partnerships (MacDonald, 2005). The education and training of the physical education teacher of the future must address these challenges and should equip teachers with the skills and knowledge and understanding to make partnerships effective. Whilst there is evidence that partnership working has not always succeeded in delivering its goals, there is little doubt that it has made a qualitative difference to pupils. The traditional conception of a teacher who works solely within the confines of the school is a vision of the past. The physical education teacher of the future needs to work with partners outside the school context in order to maximize the learning opportunities for all pupils.

Learning More

If you are interested in reading more about the background to developments surrounding partnership approaches to the delivery of PESS in the UK, the following sources provide a useful insight (Bowe et al., 1992; Flintoff, 2003; Green, 2004; Houlihan and Green, 2006). The Department for Culture Media and Sport's (DCMS) own website (www.culture.gov.uk) is a useful resource from which to access information about the UK Government's plans for sport and school sport. The DCMS/Strategy Unit (2002) policy document *Game Plan: A Strategy for Delivering Government's Sport and Physical Activity Objectives* provides a particularly useful account of the rationale behind partnership developments in school sport. For more specific publications on the role of specialist schools and their responsibility for developing partnerships with local agencies (see Bell and West, 2003; Cashbon and Walters, 2004). You may also wish to visit the website of the Institute of Youth Sport (IYS) http://info.lut.ac.uk/departments/sses/institutes/iys/index.html for useful downloads, survey materials and annual reports into the work of SSPs in the UK.

References

Audit Commission (1998) *Changing Partners: A Discussion Paper on the Role of the Local Education Authority.* Abingdon: Audit Commission Publications.

Cabinet Office (1999) *Modernising Government: Executive Summary.* London: NAO, HMSO.

DEET (2000) *Public Education: The Next Generation – Report of the Ministerial Working Party.* Victoria: DEET Publications.

DfEE (2000) *The Role of the Local Education Authority in School Education.* Nottingham: DfEE Publications.

DfES (2003) *A New Specialist System: Transforming Secondary Education.* London: DfES.

DfES/DCMS (2002) *Learning through PE and Sport.* Nottinghamshire: DfES Publications.

Donovan, M., Jones, G. and Hardman, K. (2006) Physical education and sport in England: Dualism, partnership and delivery provision, *Kinesiology*, 38(1), pp. 16–27.

Evans, J. and Penney, D. (1998) Policy, process and power. In K. Green and K. Hardman (eds) *Physical Education: A Reader.* Aachen: Meyer and Meyer.

Evans, D., Whelan, J. and Neal, G. (2002) *Best Practice in Sports Colleges.* Loughborough: Youth Sports Trust.

Garrett, R. (2004) The response of voluntary sports clubs to Sport England's Lottery funding: cases of compliance, change and resistance, *Managing Leisure*, 9, pp. 13–29.

Green, M. and Houlihan, B. (2005) *Elite Sport Development: Policy Learning and Political Priorities.* London: Routledge.

Hutt, M.D., Stafford, E.R., Walker, B.A. and Reingen, P.H. (2000) Defining the social network of a strategic alliance, *Sloan Management Review*, 41(2), pp. 51–62.

James, O. (2004) The UK core executive's use of public service agreements as a tool of governance, *Public Administration*, 82(2), pp. 397–419.

Kay, W. (2003) Physical education, RIP? *British Journal of Teaching Physical Education*, 34(4), pp. 6–10.

Kirk, D. and Gorely, T. (2000) Challenging thinking about the relationship between school physical education and sport performance, *European Physical Education Review*, 6(2), pp. 119–134.

MacDonald, I. (2005) Theorising partnerships: governance, communicative action and sport policy, *Journal of Social Policy*, 34(4), pp. 579–600.

Marshall, J. and Hardman, K. (2008) The state and status of physical education in schools in international context, *European Physical Education Review*, 6(3), pp. 203–229.

PEAUK (1997) *The Prince Philip Lecture: Physical Education Matters.* Sue Campbell, Fellows' Lecture 1997 – physical education: www.pea.uk.com/features (accessed: 15 March 2005).

Penney, D. and Evans, J. (1997) Naming the game: Discourse and domination in PE and sport in England and Wales, *European Physical Education Review*, 3(1), pp. 21–32.

Penney, D. and Houlihan, B. (2001) Re-shaping the borders for policy research: the development of specialist sports colleges in England. Paper presented at The Australian Association for Research in Education Conference, December 2001 in Fremantle, Australia.

13 Health and Safety for Learning

Peter Whitlam

Safe practice in physical education is central to successful learning and teaching in the activity. Knowledge, understanding and application of the key concepts empower pupils to manage their own safety as well as being an entitlement to learning. Teachers of physical education have a duty to be pro-active rather than reactive in relation to providing a safe learning environment. Teachers need to know the basic legal framework they operate within in their school and the importance of managing risk – the likelihood of injury – through effective forward planning and teaching of the subject. This involves applying a risk-benefit assessment in their work – in order to demonstrate that they have considered the balancing of risks without the undue danger of serious harm arising. Achieving a balanced risk–benefit decision involves the application of a series of good teaching and good organization principles. This chapter sets out the considerations that should be made to achieve such a risk–benefit balance.

Safety

Students learn about safety education through:

1. the delivery styles of the adults teaching them;
2. the school context in which they learn; and
3. increasing involvement in safe practice processes appropriate to their ages and abilities.

All students deserve high quality physical education that involves exciting and challenging experiences in a safe working environment. Involvement in their own safety also empowers them in managing their safety in future independent activity. This is often referred to as developing *risk (or safety) education* with an understanding of the risk assessment process a worthy aspect of a modern curriculum.

Safe practice in physical education is more commonly referred to as *risk management* (Severs, 2003). *Risk* in physical education can be defined simply as the likelihood of injury occurring. Managing risk effectively initially involves considering the potential safety issues relevant to the particular circumstances and deciding whether existing routines, procedures and precautions are adequate. This is the exercise of *risk assessment*. The second consideration is whether any additional procedures, routines or precautions are needed to make the situation safe. This is the application of *risk control*. Risk assessment and risk control form the concept of risk management.

The concept of 'risk' is all too often considered from a negative perspective only. However, '*risk management is about enabling good things to happen, not just preventing the bad*' (Drennan, 2008). Enjoyable, exciting and challenging physical education and school sport (PESS) experiences should be considered positively by those adults delivering lessons and sessions. Injuries occur rarely in physical education lessons and the majority of those that do occur are genuine accidents where the outcome could not be reasonably foreseen and no fault applies to the staff leading the session, as evidenced in the small number of injuries reported annually compared with the total number of pupil-days per year in physical education.

It is important to consider managing risk as the application of *good practice* and that good practice is safe practice. From this position, risk management as being '*routine, embedded and well documented*' can be more easily achieved (Shewry, 2008). Within this, *routine* may be defined as exhibiting an appropriate health and safety standard in our normal teaching processes – something described by some teachers as 'natural' because of their expertise and confidence. *Embedded* reflects consistent practice across the staff contributing to the PESS programme. *Well-documented* means having written risk assessments for PESS and documented procedures sufficient to promote a consistent standard of health and safety awareness across those contributing to the PESS programme – this is often referred to as a subject handbook or policy and guidelines for safe practice.

It is frequently stated that a key aspect of the staff role is to minimize risk in PESS, a concept promoted by the media which may lead to risk aversion or avoiding risk to avoid the possibility of injury. Unfortunately it also creates a lack of challenge, is too safe and prevents progression and student engagement occurring. In fact our task is to manage, not minimize, risk by balancing appropriate challenge with acceptable risk (afPE, 2008).

If one considers a continuum from a totally safe context to one that is dangerous then an increased likelihood of injury occurring can be anticipated as one progresses along the continuum. School staff are very good at managing risk in all aspects of their work, not simply PESS. This is manifested in the constant monitoring of situations, observing of

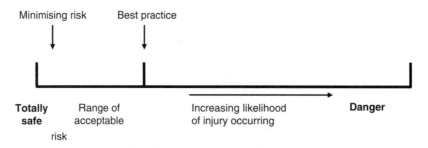

Figure 13.1 Managing risk (based on Whitlam, 2004).

students and adjusting situations within a range of acceptable risk where injury is unlikely because the pitch of the tasks set is within the capabilities of the students involved. High quality PESS, or best practice, may be defined as pitching the challenge of the students' work on the cusp of this acceptable range of risk.

There are occasions when staff recognize that a situation has progressed along the continuum to a point where injury is more likely to occur; the risk of injury is greater, where they do not feel comfortable that the experience is safe. This is, in effect, a risk assessment. They then stop the work and amend the situation to bring the context back into the range of acceptable risk – where the pitch or organization of the activity is again challenging but safe. This is an example of risk control. Across the profession this awareness and response is very evident. This is managing risk appropriately in order to achieve learning, progression and high quality.

Some colleagues deployed to deliver PESS misunderstand the expected standard of safety required, seeking to make situations as safe as possible rather than as safe as necessary. Others lack the competence and confidence to provide a learning environment where the challenge is appropriate but recognized as being within a safe context. In order for them to feel safe they actually minimize the risk by limiting the students' work to a level where the demand is insufficient to enable learning to occur; challenge is lacking and progression, excitement and high quality cannot evolve. It is important that any lack of confidence and competence by members of staff is recognized, respected and support provided to enable them to develop the confidence to allow challenging and exciting student activity to occur. In this way they will progress from minimizing risk to managing risk and be better placed to fulfil student entitlement in physical education.

All staff contributing to physical education programmes have a responsibility to know and apply the employer's policy for health and safety in physical education, inform their line manager of any issue that may harm themselves, their colleagues or others such as the students and then do what is within their power to prevent further injury arising from the problem they have reported. In addition staff have what is called a common law duty of care towards others, particularly the students, to meet expected professional standards in health and safety. This means that staff are expected to demonstrate reasonable forethought, forward planning and anticipation of what may happen in a given situation, be it a physical education lesson, an away fixture or a special event such as sports day, and to take account of the possible situations that may arise and plan to accommodate them to maintain student safety. By involving the students in this planning as a matter of policy then they will learn to become more effective in managing their own safety.

Reflection

You are about to teach an indoor physical education lesson in your school but discover that a section of the floor is wet because the roof leaks. This is an obvious slipping hazard and you must report it to your line manager/head teacher. This fulfils that part of your duty to report anything that could cause harm. You then need to do what is within your power to prevent further injury arising from that reported hazard. It is not within your power to have the roof repaired. However, you should consider a range of practical strategies to try to keep a practical lesson going.

   List as many such possibilities as you can (e.g. you could inform the pupils of the wet area – involving them in their own safety – and telling them to take care) that you may apply before deciding that it is not possible to continue a lesson.

Quality Provision

The two most significant influences on student standards and attainment are the quality of teaching and the quality of leadership and management. The same criteria can be applied effectively to health and safety in PESS.

Quality of teaching

Good teaching is safe teaching. Criteria that define and describe good teaching encompass what is required to promote challenging activity within a safe context. Time in departmental meetings is well spent when given to considering a short list of essential, basic factors in good teaching – which may be appropriately considered as 'tips for safe teaching in physical education'. Such an exercise is valuable in that discussion highlights the essential considerations when planning and delivering physical education sessions. This contributes to consistent practice across the staff and provides a clear standard of practice to be followed. Something like *ten tips* is a manageable number of issues to retain mentally and apply consistently to individual staff planning and teaching. This contributes towards developing good teaching, safe practice and a secure learning environment for the pupils. The application of any short list of essential good teaching criteria also contributes towards the development of risk education with the students, leading towards independence in safe activity over time.

Key Points

Devise your 'ten tips' for being a safe teacher of physical education. Include basic but essential good teaching criteria that you should consider in your planning and delivery of a physical education session. Refine this list by considering and improving your initial thoughts.

Such a departmental exercise is likely to highlight the following principles of good teaching in physical education that also reflect safe teaching and enable effective learning to take place:

1. A lesson format that includes warm up, the teaching and development of techniques and skills, and cool down.
2. Checking work-space, equipment and personal effects before and during the session.
3. A teaching position to maximize observation of the class at any time with regular scanning of the class when giving particular attention to a small group.
4. Using regular and approved practice, such as the content recommended in national and local resources – for example, national curriculum, local authority or national governing body of sport schemes.
5. Pitching challenge and progression according to ability and confidence.
6. Ensuring comparable student size, experience, strength and confidence are matched where weight bearing, physical contact or 'accelerating projectiles' are applied.
7. Adults not taking a full participation role in a task or game because of their greater strength and experience but taking advantage of opportunities to create and demonstrate desired learning contexts such as passing into space or creating width in attack.
8. Strict officiating in games so that the rules are applied consistently and safely.
9. Involving students in their own safety by checking their understanding, providing clear instructions and developing their awareness of risk assessment principles.
10. Thinking logically through a lesson. What could cause harm? Have I covered the likelihood of injury occurring?

Key Points

List a range of good teaching strategies you may use to provide for individual student progression according to ability. Then consider these from the perspective of safe practice criteria. Is there any difference?

Good teaching that reflects personalized learning and consideration of the principles of inclusion is also likely to demonstrate strategies of progression and differentiation, such as:

Working from:

- directed to open ended tasks;
- single to linked and on to combined or multiple tasks;
- simple to complex tasks (by providing more or less space, time, options, equipment, constraints or requirements);
- familiar tasks, environments or groupings to unfamiliar ones;
- variety in movement towards a demand for quality or technical accuracy;
- set to negotiated and on to self-determined tasks;
- individual work, with a partner and into group work involving co-operation, competition or leadership.

Or providing:

- different tasks for different students;
- different levels of information, support or intervention for students working on the same task;
- additional teacher time for some students (Dudley Local Education Authority, 1997).

The application of such strategies to aid progression also demonstrates safe practice. Giving attention to what are good teaching principles will also develop safe teaching principles – a focus that may enhance the understanding and confidence of staff in providing safe but challenging, high quality physical education. It will also contribute to the effective learning of safety education principles by the students. Such a teaching approach will educate the pupils about strategies to introduce greater difficulty, challenge and complexity in their activities and sport training programmes as they become more independent in their activity.

Reflection

Articulate your criteria for allowing any adult teaching physical education – whether a qualified teacher, coach or helper – to work alone, safely with a group of students. Do you meet your own requirements? If not then list your professional development needs in order to improve your confidence and competence to safely work alone with a group of students. Share this action plan with your line manager. Does your safety baseline match that of your colleagues?

All staff delivering physical education activities in a safe learning environment should be able to demonstrate a range of competences that address safe practice and the provision of a secure learning environment. These may include:

1. a level of expertise in the range of activities to be taught that is appropriate to the age and abilities of the students compared with the demand of the activity; this may include consideration of:
   - technical knowledge
   - knowledge of progression

- safety issues – both generic and specific to the activity
- the rules of any game being taught.

2. knowledge of the particular needs, behaviour and abilities of individuals within the group;
3. the observation and analysis skills to ensure that what is going on is safe – and if not, to implement strategies to make the situation safe;
4. good class control and group management skills to maintain safe organization and learning opportunities (afPE, 2008).

These criteria should be applied to all adults contributing to the physical education programme, whether specialist physical education teachers, visiting coaches, supply staff or others involved in physical education because statutory health and safety standards do not differ whoever is teaching the session, wherever it occurs, on or off-site and whether it is in lesson time or extended curriculum time.

Quality of leadership and management

Good organization and management of a subject contributes to establishing safe organization and management and a secure learning environment. This is particularly relevant to physical education.

Discussion

Discuss with your colleagues what you – and they – feel to be essential good organization and management factors for the department to meet in order to provide a safe working environment for the students; to provide consistent practice by all staff involved and develop confidence in the staff.

Subject leaders in physical education may find it beneficial to consider where the department sits in relation to management principles. For example:

1. Policy and procedures
   - a written health and safety policy exists for physical education and off-site sports visits;
   - written policies and procedures are reviewed regularly (annually);
   - required procedures and standards are known, understood and applied consistently by all adults who teach physical education, manage teams and lead groups off-site.

2. Roles, responsibilities and staff management
   - all staff understand the limits and requirements of their roles and responsibilities in relation to health and safety in physical education;
   - all adults teaching physical education, managing teams or leading visits are competent and confident in the areas they teach, officiate and lead;

- all non-qualified teacher status (QTS) staff are managed effectively;
- there are procedures for induction, continuing professional development and the monitoring of teaching for all staff;
- good teaching and leadership are developed and monitored.

3. Organization

- physical education programmes, fixture lists and visit objectives match the ability and confidence of teams and activity groups;
- attendance, participation and assessment records are maintained;
- equipment is regularly checked and, where appropriate, inspected and repaired by a reputable company;
- incident report forms are completed regularly and analysed periodically to monitor the number and any potential pattern of causes of injury in physical education in order to inform practice;
- health and safety is a standing item on the departmental meeting agenda as this demonstrates regular review of practice;
- incident report forms are completed regularly and analysed periodically to monitor the number and any potential pattern of causes of injury in physical education in order to inform practice;
- health and safety is a standing item on the departmental meeting agenda as this demonstrates regular review of practice.

4. Risk assessments:

- written risk assessments for physical education, sports events and visits are completed;
- risk assessments are evaluated after an event and updated periodically;
- off-site risk assessments consider and apply relevant aspects of the school's critical incident plans (sometimes known as crisis management or disaster plans).

Where departments are able to demonstrate that these or similar management principles and procedures are applied consistently within physical education then it is probable that very safe physical education experiences within a consistent learning context are offered. Such good management and organization of physical education helps create confidence and competence in the staff delivering the subject.

Subject leaders also need to make individual staff aware of a wide range of issues related to their planning and delivery of physical education sessions that have some relationship to whole school policies, organization, procedures and standards of safety. These may include:

- any implications of group size in relation to the activity and work space available;
- the level of supervision and support individual students and particular groups may need;
- group control and discipline procedures;
- application of policies such as those relating to jewellery and other personal effects;
- being fully aware of any student related medical issues;
- policies on physical contact with students;
- implementing fire, emergency evacuation procedures and other contingency plans;
- the need for particular facilities or equipment to be locked or secured when not in use;

- first aid and emergency procedures;
- reporting systems where unsafe procedures, equipment, facilities and standards are identified;
- safe storage of equipment;
- transporting students off-site.

Where individual staff are not familiar with such whole school policies and standards they are advised to enquire about them in order to be achieve consistent standards and practice across the department.

Risk Education

Staff provide safe working situations through required policies, procedures and standards as well as the manner in which they plan and deliver lessons. They may also develop student understanding of risk education and develop personal responsibility for safety by drawing attention to strategies they, as staff, employ to maintain safe standards. Three strategies contribute to establishing safe learning environments: supervision, protection and training. Supervision is provided by being present in an active role in education situations. Protection is provided through requirements and advice in situations such as personal protective equipment needing to be worn or through the setting of certain work parameters. Training includes tuition and student involvement in the safe practice issues.

All staff delivering physical education should involve the students in their own safety in a manner and style appropriate to their ages and abilities. Risk education principles (afPE, 2008) should form a continuing development of pupil awareness as they progress through their education. Examples of such principles may include a developing awareness and application of:

- Routines
- Space
- Tasks
- Equipment
- Behaviour.

Routines

Students need to be able to apply the risk-assessment process at their particular level taking into account their age and experience. In secondary schools it would be appropriate for them to consider how to recognize hazards, and progressively to contribute to making decisions about how to manage risks and maintain a safe learning environment. It is likely that they would usually be in a position to report any identified faults to their teacher but, as they grow older, they may be in situations where they need to know of other staff they can report any faults.

They need to be aware that jewellery and other adornments should always be removed before participating in activity and that any exception to this rule should be approved by a member of staff. It is also important that they are aware that they should not to use any equipment or facility without permission.

Policy

Check what your employer requires of you in relation to any form of policy concerning personal effects, such as the wearing of jewellery, spectacles, religious and cultural preferences and any other adornments. Be sure to apply any policy your employer requires as it is a whole school issue and not simply one specific to physical education.

Find out what professional associations and trade unions advise about the relative importance of cultural preferences and health and safety law.

Read the advice in afPE's *Safe Practice in Physical Education and School Sport*, 2008, pages 82, 99 and 100, concerning good practice. Remember, health and safety requirements underpin all decisions made about personal effects.

Students should know to inform staff taking the session if they feel unwell and to inform staff if they have a medical condition. This may range from the implications of having a cold to a more long-term issue such as diabetes or weak joints. They should learn and apply the principles of warm up and safe exercise as well as ensuring that taught techniques always form part of their own safe practice. Recognition that casual and careless participation may contribute to injury is a key personal responsibility. All students should also know what to do in emergency situations such as who to report to should anyone be injured, how to keep themselves safe at the site of an accident and what to do in the event of an evacuation from the premises. Taking account of reading abilities, students need to understand what signs mean and to follow the instructions, such as those for emergency exits, swimming pool rules or correct technique when using fitness suites.

With experience and proven responsible attitudes, students may progressively gain experience in participating more independently of the staff. In such circumstances they need to know how to summon staff in an emergency where supervision is remote.

Space

Students need to be aware of the importance of checking that they have sufficient space to work without placing others or themselves at risk of injury. They also need to develop an awareness of checking personal and general work space for hazards and, if necessary, report these to a responsible adult. Also, students should know not to use any facility without permission, what the safety procedures are for any facility made available to them and how to use safely any of the equipment made available to them.

Tasks

Students need to feel confident that they can, and should, ask for guidance when they do not fully understand the requirements of a task. They should never proceed with an activity if they are unclear about its requirements and outcomes. They should also develop a recognition of the importance of following guidance and instruction about how to participate responsibly. Tasks that involve taking part of the weight of a peer, such as in balancing tasks or when supporting, physical contact such as in tackling in rugby or soccer, or in activities where an 'accelerating projectile', such as a hard ball or javelin, are used should be undertaken with great care and concentration. Inappropriate peer pressure may lead to students attempting tasks in which they lack confidence in their ability to complete successfully. In such instances it is important that they feel able to express anxiety.

Students should be made aware of when and how fatigue can impair performance and put individuals at risk. They also need to know that they have a personal responsibility to then respond in order not to cause harm to themselves or others. They should also know when, and what type of, protective equipment is appropriate for a particular activity or sport; in what ways protective equipment can reduce, though never eliminate, the likelihood and severity of injury and how to judge whether an item of equipment offers genuine protection and fits appropriately.

Safety procedures and standards specific to all activities within the physical education programme require appropriate student knowledge, compliance and vigilance at all times because of the many potential hazards that exist.

Equipment

Students should learn how to manage and handle apparatus and equipment in a safe and responsible manner by being taught the correct techniques, performing under supervision and determining whether it is safe or not to proceed. In some areas of the physical education curriculum this will involve learning how to co-operate effectively as a team when setting out and putting away larger items of equipment. They should also learn how to check that equipment is safe to use, such as checking bolts, tension and wheels being retracted where relevant, and then alert staff to any observed dangers or defects. It is essential that they learn never to use any equipment unless authorized to do so by a member of staff and not to begin work until told by the member of staff.

Behaviour

PESS involves risk and requires a responsible attitude. It is essential that students learn that behaviour should be such that it does not interfere with learning and safe practice. Good behaviour is a key safety factor in physical education as distractions may lead to incidents that should be avoided.

Direct involvement in creating codes of conduct enables students to consider and establish the standards of behaviour appropriate to safe participation in activities and events. Such good practice may also contribute to developing self-discipline. They should also learn the importance of adhering to rules and conventions relevant to each activity, in order to reduce levels of risk to themselves and others. Advice relating to safe practice, whether verbal or written, should never be ignored. It is important to develop awareness that repetition and consolidation are a necessary part of the skill-learning process and learning to cope with this will help them to avoid impatience and frustration when progress is slow.

Conclusion

Safety in physical education activities is a very important learning experience for all students, in line with their age and ability. Such opportunity is brought about through the adults responsible for them creating good teaching situations from which the students can learn about safety. Working within a consistent and well organized departmental context, enabled by the use of clear policies, procedures, routines and standards, contributes to learning about safety. Involvement in their own safety in physical education helps establish a secure background for them to progress towards independence in exciting and challenging lifetime activity. Safety education is that important.

Learning More

The only publication setting out detailed guidance on safe practice principles in physical education in the UK is afPE's (2008) *Safe Practice in Physical Education and School Sport*. Part One covers general aspects such as individual needs, risk assessment, sports events, facilities and equipment. Part Two addresses the separate areas of activity in the physical education curriculum. Whitlam (2004) provides an explanation of the UK legal framework school staff operate within and summaries of over 100 cases that explain safe practice principles. Grayson (2001) provides guidance on the legal responsibilities and regulations that affect teaching, training and participation in physical education and sport in the UK, whilst Hart and Ritson (2002) is a comparative American version of the issues addressed in the UK resources described above. Dougherty (2002) is another American publication addressing injury and hazard within a wide range of physical education and sport activities within a common chapter format providing guidance on supervision, organization, teaching and environmental issues.

Fulbrook (2005) sets the safe management of outdoor activities in the context of recent cases and provides an outline of robust safety features that address typical hazards relevant to outdoor activities. Part of the 'Coaching Essentials' series, Sneyd (2006) focuses on safe practice in sport outlining all the safety issues associated with sports coaching and teaching. New and updated sections include Creating the Coaching Environment, Insurance, Risk Management, Emergency Procedures and First Aid.

Virtually all NGBs of Sport produce guidance relating to the safe organization of the activity. These are very helpful in clarifying standards specific to that activity. For example, the English Rugby Football Union produces 'Tackling Safety'; British Gymnastics produces a Code of Practice for trampolining and the Amateur Swimming Association/British Swimming produces 'Safe Supervision for Teaching and Coaching Swimming'.

References

afPE (2008) *Safe Practice in Physical Education and School Sport.* Leeds: Coachwise.

Dougherty, N. (2002) *Principles of Safety in Physical Education and Sport.* Reston, VA: National Association for Sport and Physical Education.

Drennan, L. (2008) Soap box, *News and Views, Zurich Municipal,* Autumn, p. 19.

Dudley Local Education Authority (1997) *Policy into Practice.* Dudley: Dudley Local Education Authority.

Fulbrook, J. (2005) *Outdoor Activities, Negligence and the Law.* Aldershot: Ashgate.

Grayson, E. (2001) *School Sports and the Law.* Kingston upon Thames: Croner.

Hart, J. and Ritson, J. (2002) *Liability and Safety in Physical Education and Sport.* Reston, VA: National Association for Sport and Physical Education.

Severs, J. (2003) *Safety and Risk in Primary School Physical Education.* London: Routledge.

Shewry, T. (2008) What's on the agenda? *News and Views, Zurich Municipal,* Autumn, pp. 13–14.

Sneyd, S. (2006) *How to Coach Sport Safely.* Leeds: Coachwise.

Whitlam, P. (2004) *Case Law in Physical Education and School Sport.* Leeds: Coachwise.

Part Three
Learners and Learning

Theories of Learning — 14

Rebecca J. Lloyd, Enrique Garcia Bengoechea and Stephen J. Smith

Chapter Outline

Why do we need to learn about learning theories? As long as my students are active, on task and not causing any problems, I am doing my job . . . right?

A key measure of teacher effectiveness is certainly that of student engagement. Yet engaged students need also to be learning something substantial, meaningful and long-lasting. In other words, the focus of learning, which is framed by the curriculum, needs to be considered carefully along with how things are learned, which is a process of gaining knowledge, skills and dispositions via instructional intent. Learning theories guide our considerations of what should be learned in physical education and how targeted knowledge, skills and dispositions can be best acquired by having us examine prior questions about what is worth knowing. These theories, as we shall see, help us pinpoint the kind of learning that is distinctive to physical education and the instructional means of enhancing such learning.

What Is Learning?

Before we deal with the abstractions of theory, first consider how you have learned to become physically educated yourself.

Reflection

Describe a significant learning experience from your childhood that involves the enhancement of your movement proficiency. Write a few paragraphs detailing the learning context, who was involved, how you learned, and what indications you had that you were subsequently more proficient than before.

Let us keep this self-analysis of learning in mind as we now engage with the behaviourist, cognitivist and situated learning theories as previously categorized by Greeno et al. (1996). As well as our offering of the organic perspective, which according to Davis et al. (2008), recognizes a more complex system of interactions. Each one, as summarized below carries us some way toward understanding what is at the heart of curriculum and instruction in physical education.

Key Points

1. The Behaviourist perspective relates learning to strengthened associations between stimuli and responses that result in observable changes of behaviour.
2. The Cognitive perspective equates learning with mental processing of information, problem solving and language acquisition.
3. The Situated Learning perspective defines learning in terms of the dynamic interactions that occur within a group or community.
4. The Organic Learning perspective is related to a complex, evolutionary interaction between individuals, communities and the world in which we live.

These theories, or 'perspectives' as we are calling them in this chapter, get a bit confused in practice. We rarely act as true cognitivists, behaviourists or pragmatists; instead we may borrow a little from each perspective in lesson preparations, instructional choices and assessment procedures. Behaviourism may be in evidence in the classroom management strategies used to help students stay on task as they move towards pre-set learning outcomes or goals. Cognitivism may be evident in the processing of information involved with skill acquisition (i.e. the acquiring or inputting of knowledge). Situated learning may involve creating a realistic learning context within a game or commensurate performance setting. Finally, organic or complex approaches to learning may be inferred when teachers attend to the overall maturation of the student, the class dynamics and the environmental repercussions as a whole.

At this point, you might think, 'That makes sense. Why would I need to explore these approaches to learning any further?' One reason for doing so is that you may find that you skew your lessons in terms of a theoretical preference, with 75 per cent of the time dedicated to motor skill development set up within a cognitive framework and practised behaviouristically, 25 per cent of the time spent in the authentic or situated learning contexts or game play, and little or no time teaching the organic pairings and patterns of movement acquisition that remind us of our evolutionary existence (as explored in Lloyd and Smith [2005] and in Smith and Lloyd [2006]). We hope that, by the end of this chapter, you will question the planning and delivery of physical education lessons so that you may add variety and depth to your students' learning experiences.

The following overview of the four learning perspectives is necessarily limited to what a developing physical education teacher may find helpful. Our intention is to provide you with enough theoretical information to help you reflect on your teaching practice so that you may optimize your students' learning experiences. We discuss each theoretical perspective in turn and in particular order of attending to the most salient aspects of learning to move. These perspectives are, therefore, explanatory of how physical education is taught presently and descriptive of how things might be done differently. Good theory is, in other words, a guide to best practice.

We use metaphor and symbols to simplify and thus help you remember the main categories of learning theories. Although somewhat reductionist in nature, a symbol attached to a learning perspective gives something tangible to consider when describing the learning process. It serves also to prompt some questions about the influence of certain learning metaphors on physical education practice. As Lakoff and Johnson (1999, p. 561) point out, many learning metaphors have to do with the assumption that the body is a 'mere vessel for a disembodied mind'. The metaphors that underlie certain theories of learning and that assume that one is not thinking unless using language, that thinking is akin to computational reasoning, that ideas are things to be stated, and that physical activity is the consequence of mental reasoning, need to be questioned. These metaphors need to be challenged if we are to appreciate more fully the learning that is distinctive to physical education.

The Body: A Behaviourist Perspective

The behaviourist learning perspective is most often represented by the metaphor of the 'blank slate' (otherwise known in its Latin form as the 'tabula rasa'). Within the Physical Education context, however, it seems more fitting to equate learning with the observable movements of the outer body. Like a blank page or a white board, the body may also be represented by an inanimate mass of clay that is ready to be written upon and moulded by the experiences of life that will be pressed upon it. The positive side of the blank slate assumption is that any learner can literally learn anything. Dispositions, talents, or innate abilities do not account for changes in behaviour. Basically, every student has an equal opportunity to learn as long as the connections between stimuli and responses are appropriately strengthened.

There are several behaviouristic assumptions and implications that apply to the learning context (Ormrod, 2006):

- the environment influences learning;
- learning is defined in terms of 'observable events' that can be thought of in terms of 'stimuli' and 'responses';

- the timing or 'contingency' between stimuli and responses play a significant role in strengthening associations.

One needs only to allow young children access to gym equipment without any prior instruction to realize the truth to this first behaviourist assumption! Balls, bats, climbing frames and swings stimulate children's activity in ways that challenge the teacher's ability to regain class control. Stimuli and responses need to be matched and tempered by ordering of the environment. Learning is then a planned, observable event that is the consequence of conditioning the relationship between stimuli and responses. This conditioning can be achieved through 'classical conditioning', which begins with a pre-existing relationship between an unconditioned stimulus (UCS), say meat in the case of Pavlov's dogs, giving an unconditioned response (UCR), which is salivation, and associating, for instance, the ringing of a bell with the presence of the meat. Very soon the bell stimulus produces the salivation. Classical conditioning may occur in physical education when unconditioned responses such as fear, anxiety or even extreme happiness are associated with neutral stimuli. Consider the example of picking teams. On one or several occasions, Mary is picked last for a sports team (UCS) and gets anxious when neither captain wants her on their team (UCR). The next time the teacher says, 'It is time to organize yourselves into groups', a conditioned stimulus (CS), Mary experiences anxiety, the conditioned response (CR). Generalization occurs with classical conditioning when the conditioned response spreads to another similar context, for example, when Mary experiences anxiety whenever it is time to do

Reflection

Have you experienced classical conditioning in the physical education context? Complete the following:

UCS: _____ UCR: _____

CS: _____ CR: _____

work in teams or groups in any subject or class. Fortunately as Pavlov discovered, 'conditioned responses don't necessarily last forever (Ormrod, 2006, p. 300) and we as teachers can intervene to shape positive feelings in the physical education environment.

Learning can be explained through 'operant conditioning' when teachers unconsciously or consciously reinforce student behaviours, and those behaviours increase in frequency. Formulated by B.F. Skinner, the principle of operant conditioning is: 'A response [R] that is followed by a reinforcing stimulus [S] . . . is more likely to occur again' (Ormrod, 2006, p. 301). In the physical education context, having immediate activity at the beginning of a lesson provides an example of how to reinforce the association between arriving in the gym on time or early (S) with an enjoyable movement experience (R). Reinforcers also produce negative or undesirable behaviours, such as when students put up their hands to demonstrate a skill but are never called upon. Consequently they may either stop volunteering altogether or engage in disruptive, attention getting behaviours. Praise and attention given to each and every student shape demonstrably the learning environment.

Reinforcers come in many forms. Student behaviour can be shaped by concrete objects (such as a sticker or money), social interactions (smiles, shared joy), activities (free time) and positive feedback (specific verbal praise) (Ormrod, 2006). As students get older, the contingency or timing between a behaviour and a reinforcer can increase. An older student may be motivated to work hard if free time is given at the end of a week, whereas a younger student works best if the reinforcer is immediate and tangible. Punishment, however, is not directly related to operant conditioning since it produces a decrease in the frequency of a response. If punishment is required, it can take the form of presenting an undesirable stimulus or removing a pleasant one (such as giving 'time out' from enjoyable class activity). Otherwise pleasing movement experiences can also be used as punishments, such as when push-ups or laps are assigned to disruptive students and a dislike for the prescribed activities necessarily develops. Alternatively, a 'time out' may be exactly what a student wants if the activity is not desirable.

While terms like 'athletic conditioning' are used in physical education, we need to be somewhat wary of applying behaviourist learning theory. Drawing implications from animal research may be our first clue to such wariness, especially in light of recent thinking about animal consciousness (Calarco, 2008; Haraway, 2008). Behaviourism implies that students who continue to work towards goals but are dependent on cues, feedback or rewards from the teacher, remain externally motivated. In fact, rewards to complete tasks may take away from the quality of the learning experience as students aim to 'do things quickly rather than well' (Ormrod, 2006, p. 324). If all that is recorded and rewarded in fitness testing, for example, are the quantitative data associated with numbers of repetitions or the distance covered within a set period of time, then students are not likely to develop movement quality through the enjoyment of pursuing physical activity for its own sake (Smith and Lloyd, 2007).

The Mind: A Cognitive Learning Perspective

The present day metaphor that best represents the field of cognitivism, sometimes referred to as 'mentalism' (Davis et al., 2008) is the computer as it is the most common device that represents a correspondence between the internal and external world. Actions of learning, in keeping with this metaphor, have to do with inputting, storing, processing and retrieving information. Earlier metaphors for learning within this theoretical perspective include 'sculpting, painting, writing, telegraphing, photographing or filming' (Davis et al., 2008, p. 96), but these metaphors of mimetic representation have been replaced by the computer metaphor of cerebral data processing. Learning is considered a function of a disembodied or pure mind that discounts the influence of the senses. The main principle of cognitivism is that the acquisition of knowledge is attributable to reason alone, independent of the external senses of sight, taste, touch, feel and smell (Greeno et al., 1996) and the internal senses of proprioception and kinesthesia.

Although cognitivism can be considered the exact opposite of behaviourism, stressing the processing of the mind instead of the observable actions of the physical body, these two learning perspectives are actually closely linked. Both rest on the Cartesian assumption that the mind is separated in substance and function from the physical body. The motor skill approach to learning, for example, is based on the assumption that the human body is a machine and that learning relates to the acquisition of knowledge about how to move the body efficiently, skilfully and with goal directedness (Magill, 2001). What is notably missing is any recognition of the 'physical foundations of mindfulness' and those moments in physical education when 'our body and mind come together as a unified phenomenon' that experiences itself both mindfully aware of and deeply connected to the world" (Johnson, 2000, p. 131). Call them moments of deep play, flow, peak experience, or even being in the zone. These notable experiences of physical activity are difficult to compute!

The separation of mind from body within the cognitive orientation is surprising since the roots of cognitive development theories, traced back to Jean Piaget in the 1920s (Flavell, 1998), involved explorations of children in motion, connecting with the external world. Coined 'constructivism' where 'children construct knowledge from their experiences' (Ormrod et al., 2006, p. 17), Piaget's theory describes how thought develops: first of all, from the physical, or sensorimotor stage of stimulus-response operations; second, in the pre-operational stage of initial schematic and symbolic representations; third, in the stage of concrete operations involving logical thought; and fourth and finally, in the stage of formal operations which signals adult reasoning and the capacity to problem solve and engage in abstract, hypothetical thinking processes.

Piagetian theory continues to influence physical education. The widespread advocacy of 'developmentally appropriate physical education practices for children' is premised on an understanding of development patterns and stages in all three domains (psychomotor, cognitive and affective) (NASPE, 1992; Gallahue and Donelly, 2003). A complementary perspective, the conceptual approach, emphasizes the how and the why of movement, which helps enhance the students' understanding of movement and its underlying principles. The assumption that children learn in stages, although many contemporary theorists discount a linear progression from one discrete stage to the next, indicates that children benefit from sensori-motor and concrete experiences when learning new things. We call this 'hands on learning' and it is particularly appropriate in physical education where learners need to get a feel for the touch, weight, pressure and release of passing and catching a ball before such actions are subject to the schemas and decision-making of game play.

The Community: A Situated Learning Perspective

The situated learning perspective, often attributed to Jean Lave and Etienne Wenger (1991) who describe learning in relation to legitimate participation within a community of practice, can be traced back to the Russian psychologist Lev Vygotsky. He, like Piaget, also studied cognitive development in the 1920s, but unlike Piaget's individual approach to cognitive development, Vygotsky believed that learning was a consequence of human interaction (Vygotsky, 1986). What has particular relevance for a physical education theorist is Vygotsky's assertion that action is a form of thought. Rather than localizing thought to the mind (which is often assumed to be located in one's head), he claimed that we are observing 'the real thinking of a child' when that child is engaged in the flow of activity (p. 55). With respect to cognitive development, however, Vygotsky shared the same tendency as Piaget of moving away from physical action, considering it to be 'internalized' over time and represented in language.

Lave and Wenger (1991) elaborated further on the sociolcultural approach to learning in moving away from Vygotsky's notion of internalization. They felt that a focus on internalization makes a 'sharp dichotomy between inside and outside', suggesting that 'knowledge is 'largely cerebral' and that the individual is a 'nonproblematic unit of analysis', with learning being mostly a 'matter of transmission and assimilation' (Lave and Wenger, 1991, p. 47). By contrast, learning in a situated context is defined as 'increasing participation in communities of practice' which take into account 'the whole person acting in the world' (p. 49).

Many physical education theorists have caught on to the benefits of the situated approach to learning games and sports. Researchers such as Catherine Ennis (2000) and Daryl Siedentop, Peter Hastie and Hans van der Mars (2004) promote concepts such as 'care' and 'peace' through sport education models. Low skilled students, for example, may learn by caring for the highly skilled in assuming roles that are helpful to the team such as keeping score. Highly skilled students, in turn, may care for the low skilled players by assisting them with skill development. The Teaching Games for Understanding (TGfU) also offers a situated approach to learning as it advocates learning tactics and skills within the playing of games and sports (Butler and McCahn, 2005). Within the TGfU approach, students have an opportunity to experience the joy associated with game-play right from the very beginning of a physical education lesson (Lloyd and Smith, forthcoming).

Situated learning theory thus poses some important considerations in physical education programming. First of all, it suggests that learning is essentially interactive, that it involves playing and moving with objects, with bats and balls, to music, and with other players and movers who share the space and time of the gym, the playing field, the pool or the dance studio. Becoming physically educated is very much a process of learning to move, with what is now fashionable to call 'bodily-kinesthetic intelligence' (Gardner, 1993), but in concert with others who are engaged in the communities of practice we call games, sports, gymnastics and dance. Second, these theories suggest that learning is motivated by the experience of engaging in activity that is 'autotelic'. Not merely motivated by stimulus-response connections, nor simply guided by cognitive decision-making, learning is sustained by the experience of movement itself and, particularly, by the experiences of 'flow' that are intrinsically rewarding (Csikszentmihalyi, 1990; Jackson and Csikszentmihalyi, 1999).

Reflection

Reflect on your significant learning experience and describe moments of learning that extended beyond the conditioning of a drill (behaviourist perspective) or a decision that was made (cognitive perspective). Specifically, think of a moment where learning was connected to the interaction between others, the environment, and you.

The World: An Organic Approach to Learning

The apple is a common symbol for schooling or learning. Often associated with a gift for a teacher, an apple can also represent the complex systems of interaction (Davis et al., 2008) that lead to its gestation and presence in the classroom. It symbolizes learning that does not just occur in the here and now, but is anticipated, prefigured, configured and destined to bear fruit here, there and elsewhere.

The common thread between the previously discussed 'situated learning' perspective and the 'complex' or 'organic' approach to learning, is that legitimate participation in acommunity of practice not only maintains knowledge of a repertoire shared by others, it presents 'opportunities to elaborate that repertoire' (Davis et al., 2008, p. 171). Learning, within this fourth perspective, is not only based on participation but the expansion or overall growth of the learner, community and place wherein all are situated. Knowledge is no longer a noun or a thing one must acquire (as in the cognitive paradigm), rather, 'knowing is about who you are, what you are doing, and it unfolds within interlaced sets of political, social, and environmental conditions', hence what is emphasized is the 'vibrant sense of connection among people and between humans and the more-than-human world' (Davis et al., 2008, p. 11).

The implication for learning within physical education of this theoretical perspective is that we ought not confine our interests to simply the knowledge, skills and dispositions required for playing games and sports well, or for excelling in gymnastics and dance, but that we consider much more broadly and interconnectedly our overall development as healthy, vibrant, vital individuals within expanding communities of practice and within the animate world at large. In contrast to the way curricular documents present fundamental movement skills in disconnected units, we might tap into the natural ebbs and flows of movements as they occur in organic, developmental pairings (Lloyd and Smith, 2005; 2006). Basic locomotor skills of walking, running, hopping, and skipping, for instance, might be better organized in terms of the developmental dynamics of impulsion, propulsion and resistance. The manipulative skills of throwing, catching, kicking, and so on might be better organized as reciprocated motions of sending and receiving. And the body agility skills of twisting, turning, balancing, bending, stretching might be better understood as motions that extend beyond the span of one's limbs to a connection with others and the wider world of movement possibilities.

Let us state this more simply. Beyond attending to the knowledge, skills and dispositions required for active participation in games, sports, gymnastics and dance, we can also attend to that which enlivens this participation. The complex or organic perspective on learning suggests we consider the fundamental properties of breath, balance, rhythm and feeling that animate movements within these disciplines and that bring us in touch with the animate consciousness we share with others (Sheets-Johnstone, 1999). As we depart from the mechanical learning of motor skills to create opportunities to experience dynamic patterns found within games and life, we consider cultivating vitality, energy, flow and synergy as the primary purposes of physical education (Smith and Lloyd, 2006).

The organic approach to learning not only puts us in touch with the physicality of learning, but more specifically, with the organic, dynamic nature of thought itself. No longer reduced to body objects, computers or even individuals within communities, we connect to the vitalities, flows, energies and synergies of an organic world of which we are fundamentally, motorically, kinetically and kinesthetically a part.

Reflection

Choose a lesson plan that you have recently developed for a physical education class. Analyse the planned activities and describe the theoretical assumptions you made with regard to student learning. If you were to approach the lesson from a behaviourist, cognitivist, situated and/ or organic learning theory perspective, what changes would you make?

Learning More

Other sources that delve deeper into situated (Lave and Wenger, 1991) and complex (Davis et al., 2008) theories of learning are available. There are also textbooks gearedto developing teachers that give practical examples of how theories of learning and principles of education psychology can be applied in educative settings (Ormrod et al., 2006; Ormrod, 2008).

References

Butler, J. and McCahn, B.J. (2005) Teaching games for understanding as a curriculum model (pp. 33–55). In L. Griffin and J. Butler (eds), *Teaching Games for Understanding: Theory, Research, and Practice*. Champaign, IL: Human Kinetics.

Calarco, M. (2008) *Zoographies: The Question of the Animal from Heidegger to Derrida*. New York: Columbia University Press.

Csikszentmihalyi, M. (1990) *Flow: The Psychology of Optimal Experience*. New York: Harper and Row.

Davis, B., Sumara, D. and Luce-Kapler, R. (2008) *Engaging Minds: Changing Teaching in Complex Times*. Second edition. New York: Routledge.

Ennis, C.D. (2000) Canaries in the coal mine: responding to disengaged students using theme-based curricula, *Quest*, 52, pp. 119–130.

Flavell, J.H. (1998) Piaget's legacy (pp. 31–35). In A.E. Woolfolk (ed.), *Readings in Educational Psychology*. Boston, MA: Allyn and Bacon.

Gallahue, D.L. and Donelly, F.C. (2003) *Developmental Physical Education for All Children*. Fourth edition. Champaign, IL: Human Kinetics.

Gardner, H. (1993) *Multiple Intelligences: The Theory in Practice*. New York: Basic Books.

Greeno, J.G., Collins, A.M. and Resnick, L.B. (1996) Cognition and learning (pp. 15–46). In D.C. Berliner and R.C. Calfee (eds), *Handbook of Educational Psychology*. New York: Macmillan.

Haraway, D.J. (2008) *When Species Meet*. Minneapolis: University of Minnesota Press.

Jackson, S.A. and Csikszentmihalyi, M. (1999) *Flow in Sports: The Keys to Optimal Experiences and Performances*. Champaign, IL: Human Kinetics.

Johnson, W. (2000) *Aligned, Relaxed, Resilient: the Physical Foundations of Mindfulness*. Boston: Shambhala.

Lakoff, G. and Johnson, M. (1999) *Philosophy in the Flesh: the Embodied Mind and Its Challenge to Western Thought*. New York: Basic Books.

Lave, J. and Wenger, E. (1991) *Situated Learning: Legitimate Peripheral Participation*. Cambridge: Cambridge University Press.

Lloyd, R.J. and Smith, S.J. (2005) A 'vitality' approach to the design, implementation and evaluation of health-related, physical education programs, *Avante*, 11(2), pp. 120–136.

—(2006) Motion-sensitive phenomenology (pp. 289–309). In K.G. Tobin and J. Kincheloe (eds), *Doing Educational Research: A Handbook*. Rotterdam, Netherlands: Sense Publishers.

—(forthcoming) Moving to a greater understanding: A vitality approach to 'flow motion' in games and sports. In J. Butler and L. Griffin (eds), *Teaching Games for Understanding*. Champaign, IL: Human Kinetics.

Magill, R.A. (2001) *Motor Learning: Concepts and Applications*. Toronto: McGraw-Hill Higher Education.

National Association for Sport and Physical Education (NASPE) (1992) Developmentally Appropriate Physical Education Practices for Children. Reston, VA: AAHPERD Publications.

Ormrod, J.E. (2006) *Educational Psychology: Developing Learners*. Fifth edition. Upper Saddle River, NJ: Merill Prentice Hall.

Ormrod, J.E., Saklofske, D.H., Schwean, V.L., Harrison, G.L. and Andrews, J.J. (2006) *Principles of Educational Psychology*. Canadian edition. Toronto: Pearson, Prentice Hall.

Sheets-Johnstone, M. (1999) *The Primacy of Movement*. Philadelphia: John Benjamins.

Siedentop, D., Hastie, P. and van der Mars, H. (2004) *Complete Guide to Sport Education*. Champaign, IL: Human Kinetics.

Smith, S.J. and Lloyd, R.J. (2006) Promoting vitality in health and physical education, *Qualitative Health Research: An International, Interdisciplinary Journal*, 16(2), pp. 245–67.

Smith, S.J. and Lloyd R.J. (2007) The assessment of vitality: An alternative to quantifying the health-related fitness experience, *Avante*, 11(3), pp. 66–76.

Vygotsky, L. (1986) *Thought and Word. Thought and Language*. Trans. A. Kozulin. Cambridge, MA: MIT Press.

Inclusive Teaching and Learning

Philip Vickerman

Meeting the diverse needs of all children is a fundamental goal for teachers in ensuring they develop an inclusive curriculum in which all pupils gain full access and entitlement to physical education. In addressing the full continuum of children's needs this will involve teachers working flexibly and creatively to design environments that are conducive to learning for all. In other words children who potentially may be marginalized and/or experience barriers to learning have the same rights to be challenged and progress in physical education. These principles and practices as we will see in this chapter will require a commitment to equality of opportunity and a desire to ensure learning is maximized for every child.

Introduction and Context

According to the World Education Forum (2000) adopting inclusive approaches to teaching and learning are a high priority and are rooted within the context of the United Nations (2008) promotion of 'Education for All'. The intention of such approaches is to increase the participation and learning of children who are perceived to be vulnerable of marginalization and/or barriers to learning. The World Education Forum (2000) continues that the aim of inclusive education is to eliminate social exclusion and promote diversity of opportunity for children with a particular focus upon issues of race, social class, ethnicity, religion, gender and ability. Thus according to Bailey (2005) equality of opportunity in physical education should focus upon celebration of difference and diversity amongst children that is matched by a commitment to treat people differently but fairly according to their individual needs.

Internationally, many educational authorities have adopted a philosophy of inclusion to address their social and moral obligations to educate all children and in attempting to accommodate the diverse range of needs this has led to a plethora of philosophies, policies and practices for promoting entitlement and accessibility to physical education. Norwich (2002, p. 483) for example suggests 'there is no logical purity in education', rather there is 'ideological impurity', in which no single value or principle encompasses all of what is considered worthwhile. As a result, there needs to be recognition of a range of 'multiple values' (Norwich, 2002, p. 483) through which a series of inter-related concepts, ideologies, learning, teaching and assessment practices are recognized as contributing to the removal of barriers to learning.

Creating a precise definition of what inclusive education constitutes can be problematic due to the complexity of children it refers to. Booth et al. (2000, p. 12) suggest that 'inclusion is a set of never ending processes. It involves the specification of the direction of change. It is relevant to any school however inclusive or exclusive its current cultures, policies and practices. It requires schools to engage in a critical examination of what can be done to increase the learning and participation of the diversity of students within the school locality'. In contrast Ballard (1997, p. 244) suggests 'inclusive education means education that is non-discriminatory in terms of disability, culture, gender or other aspects of students or staff that are assigned significance by a society. It involves all students in a community, with no exceptions and irrespective of their intellectual, physical, sensory or other differences, having equal rights to access the culturally valued curriculum of their society as full-timed valued members of age-appropriate mainstream classes. Inclusion emphasizes diversity over assimilation, striving to avoid the colonization of minority experiences by dominant modes of thought and action'. Consequently, whilst attempts to define what inclusion is and how it is delivered may be complex this chapter sets out to examine its relationship to physical education whilst drawing out key principles you can follow to ensure all children gain their full entitlement to a high quality education. The chapter will explore a range of learning; teaching and assessment strategies alongside examination of practical strategies for supporting the diversity of individual needs teachers are expected to support in physical education.

Focuses of Causation and Interpretations of Inclusion

The Location and Causation of barriers to learning in physical education has been subject of much debate by authors such as Fredrickson and Cline (2002), Farrell (2000) and Lloyd (2000).

In support of developments in models of inclusion Fredrickson and Cline (2002) suggest a combination of individual differences; environmental demands and interactional analyses have contributed to differing perspectives on inclusion. In relation to individual models of inclusion these view barriers to learning as being owned by the individual child. Thus if a Muslim girl cannot access mixed swimming because of her cultural and religious beliefs the problem is considered as hers rather than the schools to be proactive in responding to address her needs by offering alternative activities; facilitating single sex lessons; or enabling the child to swim in full length swimwear (see Khanifar, 2008). Another example may be where a disabled boy cannot access a gymnastics lesson because of lack of adapted equipment which is seen as a barrier that has been created by his disability rather than the school developing alternative and/or modified equipment and activities to meet his particular needs. Thus individual models of inclusion tend to advocate that barriers to learning are created by children's diversity and as such the causation of exclusion is owned by them rather than the school or physical education teacher.

According to Burchardt (2004), environmental models in contrast adopt a situation, rather than person centred focus to inclusive physical education. Cole (2008) suggests barriers to learning and access to high quality inclusive teaching and learning can only be defined in terms of relationships between what a child can do, and what a teacher must do to enable success in any given environment. Thus the limiting factor for a child being included effectively rests with the physical education teacher and school to adopt flexible approaches to learning, teaching and assessment rather than the child being expected to fit into pre-existing structures. Thus barriers to learning, teaching and assessment are considered to be created by teachers and schools lack of flexibility rather than any 'deficit' the child may bring to the activity. Frederickson and Cline (2002, p. 40) support this view by suggesting therefore that 'at one extreme then, the environmentally focused approach holds that there are no children with learning difficulties, only adults with teaching difficulties'.

Reflection

Reflect upon the quote by Fredrickson and Cline (2000) that there are no children with learning difficulties, only adults with teaching difficulties. Consider what you think the implications, strategies and challenges are for Physical Education teachers if they are to embrace this message.

In drawing the similarities and differences of individual and environmental models of inclusion together, interactional models note impossibility in separating the learning competencies of individual children from the environment within which they live and function (Booth et al., 1998). Thus models of causation and location of barriers to learning in physical education are seen as a combination of complex interactions between the strengths and weaknesses of the child, levels of support available and the appropriateness of education being provided. Thus neither environmental nor individual models exclusively describe the reality of inclusive physical education. Rather the central factor in developing inclusive physical education should be premised upon concern for high quality teaching and learning (see Rink and Hall, 2008) alongside an ability for teachers to be equipped with the necessary knowledge, skills and understanding to support a wide range of children's needs. Furthermore positive school cultures and a willingness to modify and adapt activities and environments so they are conducive to inclusive learning are crucial to the success or failure of inclusive physical education (Centre for Studies in Inclusive Education [CSIE] 2000).

Setting High Standards in Learning, Teaching and Assessment of Inclusive Physical Education

The Increasing International emphasis on inclusion was initially stimulated by the Salamanca Statement (United Nations Educational Scientific and Cultural Organisation [UNESCO], 1994) which was signed by 92 governments and 25 international organizations. It established a set of beliefs and proclamations that every child has a fundamental right to education and identified core principles of providing children with the opportunity to learn, an education system designed to take account of diversity, access to regular child centred education and the acceptance of inclusive orientation as a means of combating discrimination and building an inclusive society. The Salamanca Statement (UNESCO, 1994) has led to a multiplicity of legislation, policies, procedures and practices in different countries (see Peters, 2007; Rogers, 2007; CSIE, 2008) all of which have general focus of addressing entitlement to barrier free education.

In interpreting this statement with reference to physical education teachers are expected to establish a set of core values within their learning, teaching and assessment styles and strategies which celebrate difference and diversity. Indeed physical education particularly offers many opportunities for children to learn mutual understanding and respect for each other which fulfils many broader aspects of government citizenship agendas of fostering mutual understanding and respect for diversity. Moreover the National Curriculum (Qualification Curriculum Authority, 2007) within the United Kingdom (UK) has set out to suggest how this can be addressed via three principles of:

- **Setting suitable learning challenges:** Physical education teachers should recognize that in order to reflect diversity of children they should develop different objectives for children based upon their individual needs and differences. For example a child who has a learning difficulty may be set a task of creating a dance routine with five sequences in contrast to their non-disabled peers who may be asked to develop more (see Vickerman, 2007).

- **Responding to the diverse needs of pupils:** This places a requirement on teachers to acknowledge difference and diversity of children in physical education whilst embracing interactional models of inclusion (noted earlier) and as such modify activities as required (see Coates and Vickerman, 2008).
- **Differentiating assessment and learning to meet individual needs of pupils:** This recognizes that if physical education teachers are to set appropriate objectives and recognize children are all on a continuum of learning then they should also offer alternative methods of assessment which maximize opportunities for children to demonstrate their knowledge and understanding. For example, a child may be asked to verbally describe rather than physically demonstrate the principles of a forward roll in gymnastics if they had a physical disability.

Reflection

Review the three expectations of Physical Education teachers to set suitable learning challenges; respond to the diverse needs of pupils; and differentiate assessment and learning to meet individual needs of pupils. Consider what strategies you would adopt in order to ensure these points are addressed and all children receive their entitlement to high quality Physical Education.

As part of a commitment to establish high standards in inclusive physical education there are four basic elements that teachers should be aware impact on learning and have a particular impact on removal and/or creation of barriers to learning. These are social contexts; knowledge; the curriculum; and psychological issues. As such It is vital that teachers have a thorough appreciation of the potential impact these can have on the success or otherwise of a child's learning and development (see Bee and Boyd, 2006).

- **Social contexts** refer to the relationship between teaching and learning environments and the ideological thinking and philosophical approaches of the time such as the curriculum, school culture and the individual needs of children. Consequently in order to deliver inclusive physical education teachers must review how these factors can be addressed to maximize access to learning.
- **Knowledge** has a significant impact on the types of teaching, learning and assessment strategies used and pupil's development of their learning. For example, children have different levels of knowledge and understanding and teachers should accommodate this within every physical education lesson. Additionally physical education teachers have differing ranges of knowledge of individual needs and support should be given through training and support as required.
- **The curriculum** directs the nature and content of inclusive physical education and whole school approaches which are often required as part of statutory educational processes. This however requires teachers to make professional judgements on the interpretation of the curriculum and consideration of differentiated strategies (see Smith and Thomas, 2006) for inclusion.
- **Psychological issues** refer to the diverse range of theoretical and practical approaches that can be applied to teaching and learning. Additionally by creating or diminishing barriers to learning this can have a direct correlation with children's levels of self esteem, confidence, motivation and attitude towards physical education.

Learning to Move and Moving to Learn

According to Sugden and Wright (1998) physical education has a distinctive role to play for all children regardless of their individual needs as it does not just focus on the education of the physical, but also has social, emotional, cognitive, moral and language dimensions. Consequently, a first step in the teaching and learning process is to consider the learning outcomes of the physical education lesson. If these are not correct it immediately leads to possible barriers to learning which limit opportunities for children to gain their full entitlement and maximize opportunities to succeed in physical education. In order to address this concern learning outcomes should be developed around a focus of learning to move and/or moving to learn.

Learning to move can be considered as an intrinsic benefit of physical education and is a traditional outcome of a lesson. Here, teachers identify skills to be taught and learned by the children in a variety of contexts. This may also have a particular focus if a child has movement difficulties in which outcomes may need to be modified to accommodate this. Alternatively it may involve the use of pictures and/or videos for a child where English is an additional language in order to assist with understanding what is expected of them. In contrast, moving to learn involves developing outcomes that are based upon the results of broader experiences in physical education rather than a focus on quality of movement. Thus according to Mouratadis et al. (2008) by teachers focusing upon extrinsic benefits such as developing pupil's co-operation, empathy, team work, leadership skills and the like this can enable more pupils to access to physical education by simply changing the focus of the learning outcome for some children. For example, if a child needs to learn how to take turns or listen to the views of others this can be identified as a specific outcome for the child to work on. Another example may be where teachers introduce pupils to Kabaddi which is a traditional team sport from the Indian subcontinent. Alongside learning the rules of the game this activity could also be used to foster mutual understanding and respect of different cultures.

Developing Equality of Opportunity in Physical Education: Some Key Principles

Vickerman (2007) suggests there are four key principles to consider which will maximize the full potential of all children regardless of their disability, race, gender, cultural differences and the like. These are entitlement, accessibility, inclusion and integrity.

In relation to entitlement, the premise is to acknowledge the fundamental right of all children to access physical education and this is of particular relevance with the emergence of inclusive legislation internationally. Secondly accessibility refers to the responsibility of physical education teachers to devise strategies to ensure all pupils gain their full entitlement to the curriculum. This involves adopting flexible approaches to learning, teaching and assessment with teachers recognizing their, rather than pupils responsibility to modify and adapt activities. With reference to the third principle of inclusion teachers of physical education should start with recognition that in any class there will be a continuum of learning needs. As such teachers should work upon the premise of planning for full inclusion (Vickerman, 2007) then work backwards to alternative and/or separate activities. It is also important to recognize here though that for some children separate activities may be the best way of achieving inclusion in physical education. For example it may be more appropriate for a child in a wheelchair to take part in an alternative activity if the rest of the class are on a grass pitch. What is important here though is that the child has been consulted and is happy with any alternative offered. This links to the final principle of integrity (Vickerman et al. 2003) which suggests that whatever the nature of learning, teaching and/or assessment strategy utilized it must be of equal worth and in no way tokenistic or patronizing.

Strategies for Including Children in Physical Education

To date the chapter has established a range of principles teachers may wish to consider when setting out to include all children in physical education. We will however now turn briefly to a review of teaching and learning strategies that have been suggested by various authors (see Coates and Vickerman, 2008) to support the inclusion of all. In reviewing the diverse range of teaching and learning models designed for inclusive education they all can be simplified to three common factors. These are based around:

- **Curriculum adaptation** – Changing what is taught;
- **Instructional modifications** – Changing how we teach;
- **Human or people resources** – Looking at changing who teaches or supports adapted aspects of physical education.

Reflection

Review the three strategies of curriculum adaptation; instructional modification; and human/people resources. Consider how you would utilize these to enable children to address barriers to learning in Physical Education. You should consider this in relation to one group who may be presented with barriers to learning due to their race, disability, gender, culture, religion or class.

Practical Examples of Inclusive Physical Education

When planning inclusive physical education it is important to start from the premise of full inclusion, and where this may not be possible, consider adaptation or modification of learning and teaching activities. A central success factor for teachers is to consult, where appropriate with children and relevant professionals as part of a multi-disciplinary approach to supporting children in physical education. This enables the pupil and teachers to consider at the planning stage any differentiation that may be required whilst supporting principles of equality, and the interactional models of inclusion.

An example of this could be in games activities such as volleyball, where pupils with a special educational need may initially require lighter, larger or different coloured balls in order to access the activity. Adaptations to rules may also need to be considered, such as allowing a player with movement restrictions more time to receive and play the ball. If utilizing such a strategy, it is vital that all members of the group understand the need for such an adaptation in order that they can play to this rule during a game.

Dance activities can be adapted to assist in aiding all children's appreciation of cultural differences by teaching for example 'alokli dance repertoire' as part of a requirement of the curriculum to work co-operatively. Here particular children from western Africa where this dance form is practised will have an opportunity to learn about their cultural dances and needs whilst also educating their peers to cultural differences from around the world.

In relation to gender differences that may precipitate barriers to learning teachers should think about how boys and girls perform in physical education and whether any barriers are a product of previous limiting or encouraging factors to take up certain activities. For example, some schools may adopt traditional approaches to physical education for boys and girls whereby certain activities are restricted to one sex or the other. Thus teachers should consider how traditional activities dominated by one sex can be challenged. Girl's football for example is one of the fastest growing sports in the UK and schools should look to how they can challenge the traditional dominance of this game by boys and perhaps establish football both within the curriculum and through extra curricula activities. Another example of challenging traditional gender bias would relate to inspiring boys to take up dance. Some schools for example have established initiatives such as ABDC (All Boy's Dance Companies) to support such initiatives.

Developing a Framework for Inclusive Physical Education

This Chapter has set out to provoke thought about how physical education teachers can think flexibly and openly about the diversity of methods to minimize barriers to learning for all children. The discussion has been presented through an examination of what the philosophy of inclusion constitutes and who it refers to; examination of inclusive theories and practices; teaching and learning strategies; and establishment of core principles for inclusive physical education. The chapter now turns to the identification of an 'Eight P' Inclusive Framework (Vickerman, 2007) which encourages those facilitating inclusive physical education to take a full and detailed review of what needs to be considered to meet the full continuum of learning needs teachers are likely to be presented with in physical education.

In considering this framework the first feature a need to appreciate the **philosophy** of inclusive physical education and its relationships to basic and fundamental human rights. This requires consideration of how human rights are supported as a society through statutory and non-statutory guidance and principles of the international Salamanca Statement (UNESCO, 1994). It therefore requires those involved in facilitating inclusive physical education to understand the philosophical basis and principles of inclusion as well as buying into the notion that all children have a fundamental entitlement to learn. Consequently, if you do not get this first belief system in place the potential to realize it in practice will be severely constrained.

In order to acknowledge the philosophical complexities of inclusion a **purposeful** approach to fulfilling the requirements of inclusive physical education should be considered to initially examining various philosophical standpoints in order to gain a clear appreciation of the rationale and arguments behind inclusive physical education.

In order to achieve this you must be **proactive** in the development, implementation, and review of inclusive physical education and be prepared to work in **partnership** and consult actively with children and professionals in order to maximize an appreciation of how to minimize barriers to learning. Additionally, inclusive physical education does necessitate a commitment to modify, adapt and change existing teaching, learning, assessment strategies, policies and practices in order to facilitate full access and entitlement to the curriculum. This must be recognized as part of a **process** model that evolves, emerges and changes over time, and as such needs regular review and reflection.

Inclusive physical education is also now reflected internationally within **policy** and legislative documentation. This sets out to publicly state how agencies are going to respond to inclusive practice, whilst also being used as a means of holding people to account (Depauw and Doll-Tepper, 2000; Lloyd, 2000). Physical education teachers ultimately must however recognize the need to move policies through into their **pedagogical** practices in order to ensure they have the necessary skills to deliver inclusive physical education. Consequently, whilst philosophies and processes are vital they must in due course be measured in terms of effective and successful inclusive **practice** that values person centred approaches to the education of children.

Reflection

Review the Eight 'P' Inclusive Physical Education Framework (Vickerman, 2007) above and reflect upon how each element relates to your issues, challenges and celebrations of facilitating inclusive Physical Education. As part of this process consider the points made within this chapter in order to clarify your thinking on how you can set out to minimize barriers to learning for all children regardless of their individual differences.

Learning More

Sources to assist in developing your understanding of the context of inclusion include (Depauw and Doll-Tepper, 2000; Norwich, 2002; Burchardt, 2004; and Bailey, 2005). Additionally texts by (Fredrickson and Cline, 2002; Centre for Studies in Education, 2008; and United Nations, 2008) provide various legislative and government reviews to developing inclusive policy and practice. Some texts have been written to address learning and teaching strategies (see Cole, 2008; Mouratadis et al., 2008; and Vickerman, 2007). For those wanting to examine pupils experiences of inclusive education texts such as (Coates and Vickerman, 2008; Rogers, 2007; and Bee and Boyd, 2006) will be useful starting points.

References

Bailey, R.P. (2005) Evaluating the relationship between physical education, sport and social inclusion, *Educational Review*, 57(1), pp. 71–90.

Ballard, K. (1997) Researching disability and inclusive education: participation, construction and interpretation, *International Journal of Inclusive Education*, 1(3), pp. 243–256.

Bee, H. and Boyd, D. (2006) *The Developing Child* (International Edition). London: Pearson.

Booth, T., Ainscow, M. and Dyson, A. (1998) England: inclusion and exclusion, in a competitive system. In T. Booth and M. Ainscow (eds), *From Them to Us: An International Study of Inclusion in England*. London: Routledge.

Booth, T., Ainscow, M., Black-Hawkins, K., Vaughan, M. and Shaw, L. (2000) *Index for Inclusion: Developing Learning and Participation in Schools*. Bristol: Centre for Studies on Inclusive Education.

Burchardt, T. (2004) Capabilities and disability: the capabilities framework and the social model of disability, *Disability and Society*, 19(7), pp. 735–751.

Centre for Studies in Inclusive Education (2008) Legislation and Guidance for Inclusive Education, http://www.csie.org.uk/inclusion/legislation.shtml.

Coates, J. and Vickerman, P. (2008) Let the children have their say: children with special educational needs experiences of physical education – a review, *Support for Learning*, 23(4), pp. 168–175.

Cole, R, (ed.) (2008) *Educating Everybody's Children: Diverse Strategies for Diverse Learners*. Alexandria, VA: Association for Supervision and Curriculum Development.

DePauw, K. and Doll-Tepper, G. (2000) Toward progressive inclusion and acceptance: myth or reality? the inclusion debate and bandwagon discourse, *Adapted Physical Activity Quarterly*, 17, pp. 135–143.

Farrell, P. (2000) The impact of research on developments in inclusive education, *International Journal of Inclusive Education*, 4, pp. 153–164.

Fredrickson, N. and Cline, T. (2002) *Special Educational Needs, Inclusion and Diversity*. Buckingham: Open University Press.

Khanifar, H., Moghimi, S., Memar, S., Jandaghi, G. (2008) Ethical considerations of physical education in an Islamic valued education system, *Online Journal of Health Ethics*, 1.

Lloyd, C. (2000) Excellence for all children – false promises! the failure of current policy for inclusive education and implications for schooling in the 21st century, *International Journal of Inclusive Education*, 4, pp. 133–152.

Mouratidis, A., Vansteenkiste, M., Lens, W. and Sideris, G. (2008) The motivating role of positive feedback in sport and physical education: evidence for a motivational model, *Journal of Sport and Exercise Psychology*, 30, pp. 240–268.

Norwich, B, (2002) education, inclusion and individual differences: recognising and resolving dilemmas, *British Journal of Education Studies*, 50, pp. 482–502.

Peters, S. (2004) *Inclusive Education: An EFA Strategy for all Children*. Washington, DC: World Bank.

Rink, J. and Hall, T. (2008) Research on effective teaching in elementary school physical education, *The Elementary School Journal*, 108, pp. 207–218.

Rogers, C, (2007) Experiencing an inclusive education: parents and their children with special educational needs, *British Journal of Sociology of Education*, 28, pp. 55–68.

Qualification Curriculum Authority (2007) *National Curriculum Physical Education*. London: Qualification Curriculum Authority.

Smith, A. and Thomas, N. (2006) Including pupils with special educational needs and disabilities in National Curriculum Physical Education: a brief review. *European Journal of Special Needs Education*, 21, pp. 69–83.

Sugden, D. and Wright, H. (1998) *Motor Co-ordination Disorders in Children*. London: Sage.

United Nations Educational, Scientific and Cultural Organisation (1994) *The Salamanca Statement and Framework for Action on Special Needs Education*. Salamanca: UNESCO.

United Nations (2008) *Education for All: Overcoming Inequality – Why Governance Matters*. Oxford: Oxford University Press.

Vickerman, P., Hayes, S. and Wetherley, A. (2003) Special educational needs and National Curriculum Physical Education. In S. Hayes and G. Stidder (eds), *Equity in Physical Education*. London: Routledge.

Vickerman, P. (2007) *Teaching Physical Education to Children with Special Educational Needs*. London: Routledge.

World Education Forum (2000) *Inclusion in Education: The Participation of Disabled Learners*. Dakar, Senegal: World Education Forum.

16 Supporting Talented Students in Physical Education

Richard Bailey and David Morley

The idea that very able students need special provision has only recently been widely accepted in the UK education system, and until the early part of the twenty-first century there was no formal policy for what is now called Gifted and Talented Education. Other English-speaking countries such as the USA and Australia had highlighted the issue some years earlier. An absence of policy documents does not mean that teachers were not expected to meet the needs of such students. However, the assumption was either that the issue of high ability was not considered sufficiently important to warrant significant investment of time and money in order to develop specific guidance (compared, say, with the teaching of children with special educational needs), or that these students' needs were already being adequately met through existing approaches. Reviews by the inspection service and other central government agencies have shown these assumptions to be naïve (HMI, 1992; House of Commons, 1999). In hindsight, the need for guidance on the teaching of Gifted and Talented students is quite clear: it has long been recognized that one of the greatest challenges facing teachers is to manage the learning needs of the various young people in their classes, especially when they have very differing abilities; and the view that the most able can 'take care of themselves' is evidently wrong to anyone who has ever stepped into a school.

So, physical education teachers like their colleagues in all other subjects need to think seriously about the education of the most able. For many years they have played a somewhat unusual dual role: on the one hand, they are expected to fulfil the educational remit of the delivery and assessment of a curricular subject; on the other hand, there is a widely held expectation that physical education teachers have a contribution to make in the development of elite sports people (Bailey and Morley, 2005).

Three Problems of Talented Development in Physical Education

Gifted and talented education is a topic laden with presumptions and misunderstandings. As we have already seen teachers of physical education have some additional issues to consider. In this section we discuss three topics that seem especially relevant for those wishing to understand the subject. To some extent these topics are open to interpretation and discussion, and we certainly hope you, the reader, do talk about them with your colleagues. However, they are not matters that can simply be ignored as they impact significantly on your practice in schools.

Physical education or sport?

We have already hinted at the first problem: the relationship between talent development in sport and in physical education. To many people outside of education this is a non-issue, as their assumption is that they are the same thing. According to this view, talented students in physical education *are* those who are very good at sport, and therefore the purpose of talent development is to support future sports stars. This is a popular view among secondary teachers (Bailey et al., 2004). However, we suggest that matters are rather more complicated than this approach suggests.

Clearly, sport plays a significant part in many physical education lessons, but it has not always been this way. For many years, physical education in state schools focused on gymnastics or military drills (Kirk, 1992), and sport was largely the domain of the independent sector. By the end of the twentieth century, though, sport had secured a firm footing in all types of schools (in the UK, USA, and most other countries), and sports-based activities continue to dominate the curriculum experienced by students today (see Chapter 1).

Many academics and practitioners question this equation of sport and physical education, and suggest that a distinction needs to be drawn. In some way this is obvious as the terms are of a different character: the former describes a type of activity; the latter describes a curriculum subject, as was highlighted by the Working Party for the National Curriculum for physical education in 1991 (DES/WO, 1991):

> Sport covers a range of physical activities in which adults and young people may participate. Physical education on the other hand is a process of learning, the context being mainly physical. The purpose of this process is to develop specific knowledge, skills and understanding, and to promote physical competence. Different sporting activities can and do contribute to this learning process, and the learning process enables participation in sport. The focus however is on the child and his or her development of physical competence, rather than the activity.

The issue is not whether sport and physical education are the same things as they clearly are not. It is the extent to which sporting activities should hold centre-stage in physical education lessons. This the focus of Tinning's (1995) remarks, when he stressed the need, in his view, to reassert the 'educational purposes of physical education' (p. 19):

> While recognising the strength of sport as a public referent for physical education, I consider that our professional work will be better facilitated by reaffirming that sport is merely one medium (in physical activity) for the development of physically educated citizens. It should not be the central focus of physical education in schools. To allow physical education to be distilled to sport . . . is to sell our subject short. Certainly sport should be part of a physical education curriculum . . . but we must remember that sport is not the most reinforcing movement form for countless individuals. Sport education's null curriculum (that is what is not taught) seems to me to include as many forms of the movement culture as sport in all its forms. (p. 20)

This quotation is useful because it shows that it makes no sense to conclude that physical education teachers ought to be 'against' sport. On the contrary, most are extremely keen on it, both professionally and personally. Rather, it shows that there are potentially negative consequences of focusing too narrowly on the *content* of sports-based provision, rather than a more broad and inclusive physical education (of which sport is an important part). Figure 16.1 offers a simple set of distinctions that make things clearer.

The distinction between the two terms has been simplified to draw attention to a vitally important point: the teacher needs to be very clear about the aims of the lessons and the outcomes that are expected from them as these decisions will determine the content, character and assessment of what is taught. When we talk about Gifted and Talented Education, the issue is even more stark, as different conceptions of sport/physical education will result in different students being identified and supported.

Sport-based provision	Physical Education
focuses on the	
participation and performance	learning
of	
'sporty' students	all students
in	
out-of-school/after-school competitions	school lessons
which requires the development of	
sport-specific skills	a broad range of movement skills, including sporting skills
is assessed in terms of	
success/participation	knowledge, skills and understanding
and is led by	
sports coaches	Physical Education teachers

Figure 16.1 Distinguishing between sport and Physical Education.

Reflection

Consider two quotations:

> Australia needs tennis players who can not only hit the good shots but can run down the returns with speed, agility and fitness. We need cricketers who can make the extra run when batting and prevent the extra one when fielding because they can sprint, dive, tumble and throw well. The foundation for all of these skills is provided in the primary schools where young minds and bodies are ideally suited to rapid and efficient learning. (Pyke, cited in Kirk and Gorely, 2000, p. 122)

> The aim of physical education is to develop physical competence so that all children are able to move efficiently, effectively and safely and understand what they are doing. (afPE's National Summit on Physical Education, 2005)

These statements offer starkly different ideas of the aims and character of Physical Education. But what would a talented student be like according to the different accounts?
  Consider a class you know well.

- Which students would you select if you were working with Pyke's idea of the subject?
- Which students would you select if you assumed afPE's aim?
- Would any students qualify for both groups?
- Would any fail to qualify? Why?
- How would you assess within these two versions of Physical Education?

It is our view that teachers and departments need to discuss these issues and come to their own decisions about the place of sport within their talent development strategy for physical education. In doing so, however, they need to bear in mind that there is an expectation that they follow statutory policies like National Curricula.

Performance or potential?

It is sometimes assumed that the identification of talented students in physical education is much easier than in other subjects (e.g. Neelands et al., 2005). The argument seems to be that whilst ability in most subjects is hidden in the heads of students, ability in physical education reveals itself for all to see: the winner is the best. As common sense as this might seem, reflection will show that it is nonsense. To demonstrate this, consider two students who are equally enthusiastic about their physical education lessons: one has wealthy parents who are very supportive of her participation in physical activities, who pay for private coaching in a number of sports, who transport her to training and competitions, and who play games with her whenever they get the chance; the other student's parents do not have much money, and the little they do have is not 'wasted' on games, especially as they think that girls ought not excel at sport. Who will perform best in assessments? It is almost certainly going to be the first student, who has benefitted from considerably more investment and support. Is she more talented than her peer? From a simple observation of the way they physically perform in lessons we have no way of knowing.

Performance in physical education activities is the result of a combination of factors that form a complex system in which the whole is greater than the sum of parts. Figure 16.2 summarizes some of the elements that might contribute to talent in physical education.

These and many other factors influence the developing ability of students. To base a judgement of talent on current performance, therefore, is to mix up those things that are within a student's control and those that are not. This is why it is wise to 'to distinguish between determinants of performance and determinants of potential/skill acquisition' (Abbott et al., 2002, p. 26). Current performance can be a poor indicator of ability since it rewards factors other than talent, such as parental income and support: it heaps privilege on privilege.

One way of conceptualizing the difference between potential and performance is as follows:

Performance = Potential – Interference

(Adapted from Steiner, 1972)

In this equation, 'interference' refers to those factors that block or interrupt the development of an individual's talent. Figure 16.3 offers a brief summary of *some of the factors* that can interfere with the realization of students' potential in physical education.

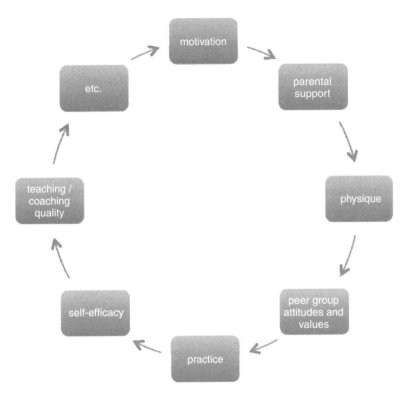

Figure 16.2 The complex system that is talent development.

Factor	Example/explanation
Gender	Many girls feel pressurized not to excel in sporting activities; many boys are discouraged from pursuing dance seriously.
Social and economic status	Engagement in some physical activities can be expensive, prohibitively so for many students.
Relative age	School years arbitrarily divide up students. This means that some in a school year can be up to a year older than their peers, a considerable advantage if physical performance is compared.
Geography	It can be much more difficult for students in rural areas to stay after school, or to travel to clubs.
Ethnicity	Minority ethnic students, as a group, take part in fewer after-school and out-of-school activities than their peers. Some students are expected to attend supplementary schools for their religion or parents' language after school.
Behaviour	Poor social skills and misbehaviour make talent identification less likely, irrespective of other abilities.
Environmental	The abilities of some students will not be identified and nurtured effectively if teaching styles and curriculum design fails to consider the range of abilities that could be exhibited in Physical Education.

Figure 16.3 'Interference' in Physical Education.

One further difficulty with performance-based assessments of ability is that teachers tend to focus on physical prowess, such as movement skills and physical fitness. Obviously these qualities are extremely important in physical education, but are not solely so. Excellence requires the development of a relatively broad range of abilities, such as social and personal skills (and this is also true in sport). The intelligent player will usually beat a less thoughtful competitor; the socially skilled team mate will be more valued that the selfish player; the player with the ability to deal with success and failure in a mature way will usually, over time, defeat those unable to deal with such experiences.

For these reasons, we are lead to conclude that while performance-based approaches have a part to play in the development of a student's talent, they should not be prioritized, as a sole reliance on them has several significant difficulties:

- They are not accurate measures of the abilities of *all* students and are particularly affected by gender, ethnicity or socio-economic background;
- They can overlook abilities that are important aspects of talent;
- They ignore students who are potentially talented, but who, due to lack of opportunity or support, are currently underachieving.

Gifted or talented?

So far we have used the terms 'gifted' and 'talented' in a rather vague way, but we now need to be clearer. Different countries and writers on the subject use these words in various ways. One popular way of dividing up the terms is that of Gagné (1991) who equates gifts with innate abilities or aptitudes, and talents as skills like sport or dance that progressively emerge from the transformation of these aptitudes through training. The English approach has been rather less logical! In one context, there is a strict distinction between the so-called 'academic subjects' (English, Mathematics, Science, History, etc.), and 'art, music, physical education, or any sport or creative art' (OfSTED, 2001), with highly able students in the former group being labelled as 'gifted' and those in the latter group 'talented'. According to another approach 'gifted' is understood to refer to the multi-ability framework of physical education (see below) and 'talented' to refer to sport, primarily focusing on the Junior Athlete Education support programme (Youth Sport Trust, 2009).

Putting aside the obvious difficulties of this way of cutting up the curriculum, it seems that physical education, once again, has an unusual position. Our advice is to be aware that different groups use their own terminology and not get over-concerned with languages games: it is more important that teachers offer their students a high quality learning experience than they invest time getting the terms right! For the purposes of this chapter we will simply refer to talented students (and assume the reader remembers that we include the different types of abilities that are expressed in physical education).

Now we need to move on to more practical matters, such as how to identify and support gifted and talented students in physical education.

Who Are the Gifted and Talented in Physical Education?

The two most common criteria for identifying talented students are current performance and ability in specific sports (Bailey et al., 2009). As we have seen, both of these approaches have their merits but also their limits. There are also practical questions, such as 'if your talent identification strategy focuses on sports performance, which sports will you select?' Assuming that there is a limited amount of time and money there are two ways of responding to this question: either select a small number of sports and focus support towards the students who excel in them, or concentrate on the generic, shared abilities that underlie all sports and physical activities. Our approach has been to focus on what we believe to be the core abilities of physical education (Bailey and Morley, 2006; Morley and Bailey, 2006). In formulating our list of abilities we asked 'what abilities are developed (or are claimed to be developed) in physical education?' Over time we came up with the model presented in Figure 16.4.

These abilities translate into practice and career outcomes as follows (see Figure 16.5).

Our suggestion is that students can be recognized as talented when they demonstrate high-level ability within the full range of physical education contexts, or have the potential to do so. Specifically, we suggest that talented students excel in one or more of these

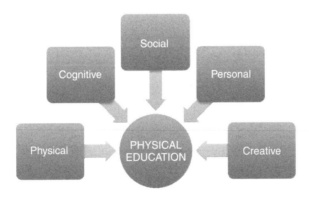

Figure 16.4 Physical Education abilities (commonly termed as 'The Multi-abilities' framework).

Ability	Definition	Possible outcomes
Physical	Often understood as skill or fitness related ability, this describes the pupil who has specific physical ability associated with high-level physical performance. A pupil with high levels of physical ability may exhibit excellence in stamina, speed, reaction, flexibility, co-ordination, etc.	• High levels of fundamental movement ability • Elite performers • High marks within practical components of examination PE
Creative	A 'style' of intelligence with a pupil displaying alternative responses to set stimuli, a broad analysis vocabulary and innovative tactics and skills.	• Innovative game tacticians • Problem solvers • Choreographers
Cognitive	The pupil's ability to transfer skills, concepts and applications between and within activities demonstrating a superior awareness of the influence of space in terms of positioning and dominance. A high level of understanding of key principles of sports and an ability to present this effectively.	• Teachers • Coaches • High marks within theoretical components of examination PE
Personal	Pupils with a high level of intrapersonal ability are well-motivated and have a constructive approach to achieving their goals. They will also regulate their own learning, set themselves goals and practice hard in their own context (coaching, leading or playing). A well-motivated pupil of average ability may be more successful than a de-motivated pupil of higher ability.	• Elite performers • Teachers • Coaches • Success within examination PE
Social	The pupil's ability to interact with others, demonstrating excellent communication skills and strong leadership qualities within a range of environments. An interpersonal deficiency may also exist in some pupils whereby they are unable to fulfil their potential as a result of the deficiency, for example, by not being able to relate to team members.	• Elite performers (particularly in team environments) • Coaches • Teachers • Expedition leaders

Figure 16.5 Physical Education abilities (based on Morley and Bailey, 2006).

abilities. Alternatively, they may give insights that, if offered sufficient support, they *could* excel. It is very likely that students will exhibit relative strengths and weakness in these areas, and this is valuable information for the teacher as it shows the domains in which individual students need more challenge and those where more structured, remedial support is necessary.

Planning Activity

Your assessment of a class reveals four students with exceptional ability in certain aspects of Physical Education.

1. Imogen is the youngest student of her year group, and is also a later physical maturer, so she is much smaller than most of her peers. Yet she is extremely motivated and determined in Physical Education lessons, and invests much more time in and out of lessons in developing her skills.
2. Morgan has reasonably strong physical skills, but he is also a great leader and coach, able to bring out the best of others.
3. Zara has very well-developed movement skills, and high levels of fitness. However, she does not perform well in a team as she is intolerant of what she takes to be the weaknesses of her team-mates.
4. Madeleine is average physical ability, but has a great tactical and creative mind for games. She can work out strategies much quicker than her peers, and can 'see' opportunities that others miss.

Using the Multi-Abilities Framework explained above, plan strategies for meeting the needs of these four very different students.

How will you differentiate your teaching to challenge them in their areas of strength?

What will you do to address their weaknesses?

If these students were in your class, would you identify all, some or none of them as talented in Physical Education? Why?

For more practical ideas on how to establish strategies for meeting the needs of these children, you might want to visit http://gifted.youthsporttrust.org, and select the 'Gifted in PE' tab.

Identifying Talented Students

Identification is the most complex and problematic area of gifted and talented education (DfEE, 1999; OfSTED, 2004). For example, Freeman (1998, p. 4) suggests, 'Each method of identifying the very able distinguishes a somewhat different group of children, with possibly different consequences for their self-concepts and education'. For this reason it is very important that opportunities to share issues surrounding the identification process are taken to ensure equitable practice throughout the process.

If it is accepted that talented children in physical education may possess high levels of ability in one or more areas then it is important that identification strategies are used that reflect this principle. Identification strategies in physical education can be grouped into three broad categories, as shown in Figure 16.6 below.

Using multiple identification criteria ensures a diverse talent cohort, which reflects the nature and scope of physical education more accurately than the purely performance-based identification procedure conventionally found in sport. Many of the simplest yet more suitable identification strategies lie at the heart of good generic teaching practice, such as formative assessment and differentiation. However, it may be the case that such generic strategies

Category	Explanation	Examples
Holistic observation	assess overall performance or target a cluster of core abilities at the same time	differentiation, formative assessment
Activity-specific measures	assessments of performance in different activities	Ability to outwit opponents, replicate actions within specific activities, e.g. games, athletics
Ability-specific strategies	focus on the assessment of an individual ability that underlies participation and performance in Physical Education contexts (physical, social, personal, cognitive and creative)	creativity tests, social capability through Sport Education (see case studies later in this chapter)

Figure 16.6 Categories of identification strategies.

only provide a broad-brush portrait of a pupil's ability and achievement so at some stage of the process there may be a need to focus on specific abilities as part of a more detailed assessment of that pupil's talent.

Providing for Talented Students

As with all inclusive approaches to teaching, meeting the needs of talented learners in physical education requires the parameters of existing teaching practices to be broadened. It is not surprising, then, that the following section on 'provision' has explicit parallels with 'best practice' principles of teaching. This viewpoint is important as provision for talented students is not something that is additional to existing teaching but is simply an aspect of provision with a different focus. This provision needs to offer opportunities for everyone to experience challenge and be stretched and must also enable a continuous cycle of identification–provision–evaluation–identification to be maintained.

There are two broad ways in which we can provide for talented students: *enrichment* and *acceleration*. The following sections discuss the key differences to these approaches and the case studies in Appendix G offer examples of how schools have adopted these in practice.

Enrichment

English school inspectors (OfSTED, 2004) reported that whilst certain methods of provision for talented pupils in physical education such as mentoring were effective, there remained a need to develop additional approaches that have mainstream curricular impact. Similarly, recent studies have found that the majority of strategies used to provide for talented pupils in physical education existed in extracurricular settings, few of which had a direct impact on mainstream curricular experiences of the talented pupils (Bailey et al., 2005; Tremere et al., 2005).

Enrichment is a process whereby an existing learning environment can be enhanced through the use of additional and often creative resources and teaching approaches designed specifically to enhance talented students' learning whilst providing equitable opportunities for all learners. A useful way to understand the ways in which enrichment can be used is to consider Renzulli's (1977) enrichment triad model.

In many respects this approach facilitates the whole talent development process from identification through to provision and as such provides an excellent tool for assessing potential outside of other structured identification systems. An example of how this three-tiered model could be used in a physical education lesson to effectively challenge talented pupils is given below.

Type 1 enrichment – inspire

At this level, students are stimulated by a theme and this is fuelled by involvement in a wide range of activities that offer further engagement. For example, in a lesson focusing on outwitting opponents the theme could be centred on beating a player in an invasion game, with skills such as feinting and dummying, or drawing a player to create space being used in a range of tactical situations and with a diverse range of equipment. Activities could be stimulated by task cards, video footage, magazines, etc., but would remain within the structured time of the lesson. At this stage recognition of talent from the multi-ability framework (in particular social ability) would be noted to guide future learning opportunities.

Type 2 enrichment – innovate

Talented students may now require specific skills to pursue their level of understanding more effectively. Using traditional approaches progression from Type 1 activities would see students continue to develop technical skills related to a specific sport. Effective enrichment would entail students' learning experiences being driven by their preferred involvement in a range of roles and responsibilities and a deeper understanding of the learning associated with engagement in tasks. In this case, this would involve the selection and development of a range of activities related to outwitting opponents by sub-groups of students who have been given access to a range of materials and resources to research in their own time.

Type 3 enrichment – initiate

Groups formalize their interest in a particular learning activity, and some groups are given the opportunity to present their ideas to the rest of the group for review. Some talented students may feel able to follow their experiences at Type 1 and Type 2 activities to continue these enrichment activities in their own time and possibly deliver their ideas to other groups, both within and beyond school.

This approach suits the multi-dimensional aspect of talent development in Physical Education very well as it allows pupils to fulfil a variety of roles within a common task.

Differentiated Practices

Differentiation is not only at the heart of inclusive and effective teaching but it is also a central feature of provision for talented students in physical education. The following diagram explains a model of differentiation that has been refined and developed to advance the traditional 'outcome' and 'task'-based differentiation approach, and in doing so presents an excellent vehicle for explaining the potential for differentiated, enriching talent development practices:

Through this model we can begin to map out some of the underlying principles of provision for talented pupils in physical education.

Differentiation by organization

Talented students often like working with peers with similar abilities as it gives them opportunities to operate at a higher level and extends their expectations of themselves and others. Mixed ability groups are the norm in physical education classes, but there is an obvious danger when this teaching targets the ability of the majority of the group (Benn and Chitty, 1996). Ability grouping is, therefore, a useful strategy as part of differentiated provision. There is research evidence showing that all students can benefit from a well-planned ability-grouped session (Freeman, 1998). More recent research has supported this finding, but stressed that the key factor in its success was the learning climate generated by the teacher (Bailey et al., 2008).

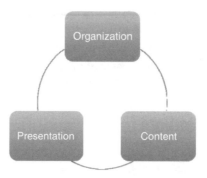

Figure 16.7 Bailey's model of differentiation (Source: Bailey, 2001).

Decisions regarding grouping should be made on the basis of the learning needs of the students and consequently such decisions will never be made in the long-term; there will always be a need to review and evaluate the grouping of students in response to their learning in order to enhance their learning experiences and this must be seen as a fluid and responsive process (see Figure 16.8).

Year grouping systems	Advantages	Disadvantages
Mixed ability	Talented pupils can be used to demonstrate and coach less able pupils	• Employing a range of practices to suit a wide range of needs is difficult • Level of delivery is often aimed at children with average ability
Streaming	Lessons can concentrate on the cognitive dimensions of the subject area and prepare for examination PE more effectively	• Although PE provides for pupils with high academic ability, abilities other than those recognized within academic subjects will not be used as primary indicators of talent
Setting by ability in PE	Assessing level of appropriate tasks and challenge is easier and pupils work at an appropriate pace for their own needs	• Generally based on current performance and therefore limited in recognizing potential • Some baseline indicators of talent may only cover certain activity areas • Potential for negative 'labelling' effect on talented group and lower sets
Setting by a single or limited number of specific activities (e.g. games)	Within the specified activity area talented pupils have the opportunity to work with other pupils of similar ability	• When the curriculum changes to other activity areas than the one used to initially group pupils, the levels of ability within the group are wide ranging
Class grouping systems	**Advantages**	**Disadvantages**
Friendship groups	Pupils are more likely to understand the strengths and weaknesses of others within their group	• Potential for talented pupils to become distracted and stray from the task
Randomly selected groups	Allows opportunities for talented pupils to develop as effective communicators and readily adopt roles in unfamiliar environments	• Does not allow for selection by ability and therefore raises issues related to appropriate challenge for all pupils within the group
Ability groups	Differentiated practices and tasks can be targeted more specifically at certain groups	• There is potential for lower ability groups to be 'left behind' and this may have implications if re-integration is to be considered

Figure 16.8 Advantages and disadvantages of differing grouping strategies with talented students in Physical Education (adapted from Morley and Bailey, 2006).

Differentiation by presentation

Teaching style

The use of a particular teaching style will have an enormous impact on the potential for talented students to access high quality learning experiences. Mosston and Ashworth (1986) developed a teaching spectrum which maps out teaching styles ranging from command style to discovery and the adoption of a range of these styles will inevitably challenge talented students effectively and prevent boredom within lessons (see Chapters 7 and 9).

Questioning

Many of the above responses may require some form of subsequent questioning to allow pupils the opportunity to elaborate on their initial thoughts or movements and also to develop their depth of learning. Open-ended questions that stimulate thinking and concentrate on process as much as product are particularly useful here, as are those that arouse curiosity through the use of probing questions; using 'why?' as a precursor to a question is as important as the question of 'how?'.

Differentiation by content

As talented students will often progress through a series of tasks at a faster rate than their peers it is appropriate to consider the most suitable level and amount of content necessary to stretch and challenge them effectively. When considering the notion of suitable content to match the individual's needs 'more' may not always be better. In this regard it may seem appropriate to accelerate talented students' learning by using material from later Key Stages of the National Curriculum or indeed by allowing them to access the different levels of examination physical education at an early stage. Whilst this may be appropriate for some students, the increase in the pace of delivery in this way presents a danger that provision will lack depth leaving higher order thinking skills underdeveloped (Eyre, 2001). This sort of 'content acceleration' needs to be treated with caution, however, as the quality of learning experiences should always be used as the primary factor (Hymer and Michel, 2002).

As already discussed, when some children are working at levels significantly beyond that of their peers the organization of curricular content can become problematic. The pace of delivery is another important aspect of ensuring quality provision for talented pupils: if the pace is too fast and pupils experience limited success, students may become frustrated and anxious about their lack of progression. Conversely, if the pace is too slow they may become frustrated and it is this type of environment that could cause talented pupils to become disaffected from the physical education altogether.

Teaching Smarter

Teachers need to explore methods of stimulating learning in different ways within lessons in order to respond to the distinctive needs of talented pupils and to help them thrive. The development of these teaching skills will not happen by chance and requires specific intervention. Such interventions could consist of:

- opportunities to 'team teach' talented pupils and discuss outcomes and future intentions;
- shadowing teachers who are more experienced in providing for talented pupils in physical education;
- exploring ways in which existing planning can be modified to cater for talented pupils more effectively;
- standardizing evidence of talented behaviours with colleagues (e.g. video, records of assessment);
- access to working groups established to evaluate talent development practices;
- exploring pathway development opportunities for talented pupils in physical education to step into sport, using a range of roles and responsibilities.

Talent Development in Physical Education: A Whole School Approach

The English Quality Standards for physical education provide the most comprehensive guidance available for the identification of and provision for talented pupils in Physical Education and sport and act here as a suitable way of summarizing the key aspects of this chapter (http://gifted.youthsporttrust.org/page/peqs/index.html). The Quality Standards provide a series of statements of outcome that reflect different degrees of good practice, from requisite (or basic) to exemplary. These statements are supplemented by strategies and tools that can help local authorities and schools progress towards exemplary practice. They are based on ten themes, offering a personalized learning framework:

1. Identification
2. Subject knowledge
3. Learning and teaching
4. Planning and setting expectations
5. Assessment for learning
6. Social and emotional needs
7. Classroom ethos and climate for learning
8. Resources
9. Parents, carers and the wider community
10. Monitoring and evaluation

The Quality Standards are differentiated to support development at different levels for schools and pupils. This framework affords an understanding of talented development practices from the differing perspectives of those involved and suggests practical approaches to ensure ongoing improvement. The Quality Standards provide a benchmark of existing practices, through self-review, and it is important that once this review is complete that the ethos and underlying principles of an approach is assimilated into a series of working practices that can be shared and owned by the whole department. These practices could otherwise be known as the 'principles of policy' and the four key principles of policy for talent development in physical education are:

1. an educational approach to talent development in physical education;
2. identification and selection;
3. teaching and provision;
4. professional development.

In each section reference is made to departmental responsibilities and also how students can be actively engaged in the talent development process.

1. An educational approach to talent development in physical education

The department:

- ensures that talent development policy for physical education is embedded within physical education and whole-school Gifted and Talented policies;
- is fully aware of the distinctive nature of physical education, and ensures that talent development in physical education maintains its educational focus;
- collaborates productively with a range of key partners in the design and implementation of talent development programmes.

Pupils:

- recognize that physical education talent development policy and practices are part of a whole-school Gifted and Talented Education programme;
- are fully aware of, and involved in, physical education talent development policies within their school, and understand how these policies impact on their physical education and general school experiences.

2. Identification and selection

The department:

- is explicit about the expectations of pupils aspiring to be identified as talented in physical education;
- devises/formulates strategies to identify diverse abilities, in order to provide students with opportunities to reveal strengths in a variety of domains;

- organizes opportunities for sharing experiences and moderating the talent identification process;
- monitors talent cohort composition to ensure equitable identification practices are taking place including disabled pupils, pupils' socio-economic status, special educational needs or medical conditions.

Pupils:

- are fully aware of the strategies employed to identify talent in physical education;
- are identified for their abilities across a wide range of physical education contexts;
- assess and nominate themselves and their peers in a range of environments to contribute to the talent identification process.

3. Teaching and support

The school ensures that:

- curricular provision is adapted, modified or replaced to meet the distinctive needs of talented pupils in physical education;
- a portfolio of evidence is gathered during identification to inform and direct the provision process;
- the focus of provision in schools for talented pupils in physical education is firmly located within curricular physical education, and reflects NC requirements.

Pupils:

- are fully aware of their strengths and areas for development, and the contribution provision strategies can make to this development;
- engage in a structured programme of activities in which they work alongside pupils with gifts and talents in physical education and other subject areas;
- are offered opportunities to discuss the impact of their talents on their personal lives with mentors and the physical education Gifted and Talented co-ordinator.

4. Professional development

The school:

- uses increased opportunities for pupils as a success criteria for the evaluation of the impact of professional development activities;
- collaborates with other schools and national bodies to remain informed of current initiatives related to talent development in physical education;
- organizes a range of ongoing subject-specific professional development;
- ensures that physical education staff are all involved in the identification of and provision for talented pupils in physical education;
- provides a comprehensive and needs-based professional development programme for all teachers and adults-other-than-teachers involved in the development of talented pupils in physical education.

Conclusion

Talent development is an exciting opportunity for teachers to adapt their skills to meet the needs of an often-overlooked group of students. It is important to remember, though, that the great majority of these skills are based on existing good practice. Flexibility, differentiation and creativity are key, and so talent development presents a great opportunity for teachers to improve their practices for the benefit of all students. As was mentioned in this chapter, the teacher's ability to generate and maintain a positive learning climate will make the difference between a programme that supports just a few students and one that supports all. In Renzulli's (1998) memorable phrase, 'a rising tide lifts all ships'.

Learning More

To date, the only book-length treatment of the topic of gifted and talented education related to physical education is by Morley and Bailey (2006). The theoretical background and rationale for recent developments is presented in Bailey and Morley (2006). The Youth Sport Trust has a useful website that is based on the Bailey-Morley model of talent development: http://gifted.youthsporttrust.org/. Create development (www.createdevelopment.co.uk) offer an excellent multi-ability based resources for teachers and coaches that aim to accelerate the abilities of children. An online self-assessment tool named the Accelerating abilities wheel is also offered as a way of monitoring and tracking student's development within the multi-ability context. Most general texts of 'G&T' are very poor when it comes to physical education, and are best avoided if your interest is specifically with this subject. However, Joan Freeman's personal website (www.joanfreeman.com) contains some useful (and free) resources, including an account of her 'Sport Approach'. By far the most comprehensive review of research into general Gifted and Talented Education is Bailey et al.'s (2008) report. Another website with useful resources, this time specifically focusing on physical education, is www.richardbailey.net.

References

Abbott, A., Collins, D., Martindale, R. and Sowerby, K. (2002) *Talent Identification and Development: An Academic Review*. Edinburgh: sportscotland.

afPE (Association for Physical Education) (2005) National Summit on Physical Education, London, 24 January 2005. Available from: www.afpe.org.uk/public/downloads/national_summit.pdf (accessed: 20 May 2009).

Bailey, R.P. (2001) *Teaching Physical Education – a Handbook for Primary & Secondary School Teachers*. London: Kogan Page.

Bailey, R.P. and Morley, D. (2005) Talent identification and provision in physical education – a strategic approach, *British Journal of Teaching Physical Education*, 35, pp. 41–44.

—(2006) Towards a model of talent development in physical education, *Sport, Education and Society*, 11(3), pp. 211–230.

—(2007) *Physical Education Quality Standards for Talent Development*. Loughborough: Youth Sport Trust.

Bailey, R.P., Morley, D. and Dismore, H. (2009) Talent development in physical education: a national survey of policy and practice in England, *Physical Education and Sport Pedagogy*, 14, pp. 59–72.

Bailey, R.P., Pearce, G., Winstanley, C., Sutherland, M., Smith, C., Stack, N. and Dickenson, M. (2008) A systematic review of interventions aimed at improving the educational achievement of pupils identified as gifted and talented. Report. In: *Research Evidence in Education Library*. London: EPPI-Centre, Social Science Research Unit, Institute of Education, University of London.

Bailey, R.P., Tan, J. and Morley, D. (2004) Secondary school teachers' perceptions of identifying talented pupils in physical education, *Physical Education and Sport Pedagogy*, 9, pp. 133–148.

DES (Department of Education and Science)/Welsh Office (1991) Physical Education for Ages 5–16: Proposals of the Secretary of State for Education and the Secretary of State for Wales. London: DES.

Gagné, F. (1991) Toward a differentiated model of giftedness and talent (pp. 65–80). In N. Colangelo and G.A. Davis (eds), *Handbook of Gifted Education*. Boston, MA: Allyn and Bacon.

HMI (Her Majesty's Inspectorate) (1992) *The Education of Very Able Children in Maintained Schools. A Review by HMI*. London: HMSO.

House of Commons (1999) Education and Employment Committee, third report, *Highly Able Children*. London: HMSO.

Kirk, D. (1992) *Defining Physical Education: The Social Construction of a School Subject in Postwar Britain*. London: Falmer Press.

Kirk, D. and Gorely, T. (2000) Challenging thinking about the relationship between school physical education and sport performance, *European Physical Educational Review*, 6, pp. 119–134.

Morley, D. and Bailey, R.P. (2006) *Meeting the Needs of Very Able Pupils in Physical Education and Sport*. London: David Fulton.

Neelands, J., Band, S., Freckley, V. and Lindsay, G. (2005) *Hidden Talents: A Review of State Supported Provision and Policy for Talented Pupils in England*. Coventry: National Academy for Gifted and Talented Youth.

OfSTED (2001) *Guidance to Inspectors – the Identification and Provision for Gifted and Talented Pupils*. London: Office for Standards in Education.

Steiner, I.D. (1972) *Group Processes and Productivity*. New York: Academic Press.

The Youth Sport Trust (2009) Talented in Sport. http://gifted.youthsporttrust.org/ (accessed: 9 July 2009).

17 Listening to Pupils' Voices

Ann MacPhail

Chapter Outline

Research has demonstrated that pupils enjoy, are motivated by and strengthen their self-esteem and respect by being consulted about their school experiences, and welcome the opportunity to share ideas that may help them to learn more effectively. This chapter reports pupil voice and consultation discussions before contextualizing the discussion in school physical education, recognizing the need to explore links between young people's voices in and beyond school.

Introduction

If we view the world through the eyes of our students and hear the messages embedded in their actions, we will learn things we never knew we did not know. There seem to be some consistent messages from our students – messages about the content of the curriculum, their value perceptions, and the meaningfulness of their experiences.

(Lee, 1997, p. 274)

There may be a tendency to underestimate the extent to which pupils care and are perceptive about their educational progress. However, numerous studies and the quotation above provide evidence that pupils enjoy, are motivated by and strengthen their self-esteem and respect by being consulted about their school experiences and welcome the opportunity to share ideas that may help them to learn more effectively. This can convey to pupils that they are legitimate members of the schooling system, and acknowledge that a worthwhile school experience relies on the pupils and teacher informing each others' learning. That is, the teachers' practice of teaching is integrated with and through pupil consultation and subsequent participation.

Physical education teachers strive to provide pupils with authentic experiences that meet their changing needs and interests, with the ultimate goal being to encourage young people to be more physically active and to adopt a healthy lifestyle. It is therefore vital that teachers not only understand how pupils perceive Physical education but how values and beliefs can inform the development of effective practice in Physical education (Brooker and Macdonald, 1999). The way in which pupil voice can contribute to the construction of the Physical education curriculum in partnership with teachers (Glasby and Macdonald, 2004) is vital in providing authentic and meaningful learning experiences.

Reflection: Informing Authentic Learning Experiences in Physical Education

After reading the extract below from Luke, a 13-year old boy with Asperger Syndrome, consider how, as a teacher of physical education, you could begin to construct a physical education teaching and learning environment that would allow Luke to be authentically involved in physical education along with his peers in the class.

> Please realize that making someone do a team sport is not suddenly going to make him or her become sociable and co-ordinated. In fact it is a pretty daft idea to think that anything at all is going to make an AS [Asperger Syndrome] person suddenly have no difficulty with social interaction. That is like saying that if a blind person holds a book in front of their nose long enough they are going to suddenly be able to see! Maybe if you are still in doubt, you could put in a set of ear plugs, wear a pair of goggles and try a team sport whilst only allowing yourself to catch or kick the ball with the hand or foot that you are not used to. This is what it feels like all the time for us. It's very difficult isn't it?! (Jackson, 2002, p. 132)

This chapter reports pupil voice and consultation discussions before contextualizing the discussion in school physical education, recognizing the need to explore links between young people's voices in and beyond school. In 1989 the United Nations General Assembly adopted the Convention on the Rights of the Child, which incorporates children's (under the age of 18) civil and political, social, economic and cultural rights and their rights to protection. Fundamental to the rights of young people is for their opinions and views to be heard and considered and to have a say in matters affecting their own lives (Article 12 of the Convention). A number of national government organizations (Children and Young People's Unit in the UK and the Children's Rights Alliance in Ireland) have formally committed to uphold the Convention and actively encourage young people to become more formally involved in their own lives.

Defining 'consulting pupils' and 'participation'

This chapter refers to the working definitions for the terms 'consulting pupils' and 'participation' promoted by Rudduck and McIntyre (2007). 'Consulting' between teachers and pupils, and among pupils, about their experiences with teaching and learning in school is a way to converse about what learning is like from the pupils' perspective. 'Participation' develops such consultation with a view to strengthening pupils' opportunities for decision-making, investment and participation in schooling, in turn hoping to increase their sense of involvement in the school as a member of a learning community. It is not simply listening to pupils' voices in response to whether they understand the content but rather increasing our level of participation and engagement with them and responding to their perspectives. In short, explicitly seeking pupils' perspectives and taking full account of these as we, as teachers, strive to provide more effective learning opportunities for all pupils through the organization of schooling, pedagogical practices and relationships between teachers and pupils. Research into such participation and the impact of pupil consultation on teachers' practices and their use of pupils' ideas is becoming increasingly more prominent (see student voice Special Issues of *Educational Review* 2006 [vol. 58] and *Forum* 2001 [vol. 43] for related research).

Reflection: Pupil Evaluations of Learning and Teaching

Pupils provide input and considerations for Physical Education teachers regarding the effectiveness of the physical education curriculum, quality of teacher instructional methods and how to utilize pupil voice in the gym and sports hall. A sample of prompts (School Change Collaborative, 1997) that can be presented to pupils to initiate discussion between pupil and pupil and teacher and pupil on young people's current experiences of teaching and learning include:

- Does the teacher understand the pupils' point of view?
- Does this teacher seem to care whether pupils learn?
- Does this teacher behave differently toward pupils?
- Has this teacher been helpful to you in your learning efforts this year?
- Does the teacher usually know what he/she is talking about?
- Does the teacher give pupils the opportunity to confirm and get a firm grasp of what they have learned?
- Is the teacher enthusiastic about the class?

Once discussion of responses to the prompts has taken place the challenge is then for the teacher and pupil to co-construct more meaningful learning and teaching experiences, most likely through further discussion or through a task similar to that noted under the reflection boxes titled 'Involving students in curriculum design and development'.

A number of typologies convey the increasing levels of pupil participation and engagement in consultation. As McMahon (2007) explains, these typologies of pupil participation tend to rank projects by means of a 'ladder of participation', meaning that the higher the rung on the ladder the greater the level of pupil participation and involvement. Fielding's (2001) four-fold typology of pupil engagement links closely with such typologies, denoting increasing levels of reciprocity from 'students as data sources', to 'active respondents', to 'co-researchers' to 'researchers'. Fielding (2001) maps each level with the essential teacher and pupil role and teacher engagement with pupils. Treseder's (1997) model avoids a ladder of participation layout by placing 'degrees of participation' at the centre of his framework with opportunities for involvement placed equidistant from the centre. Such a typology acknowledges that, rather than a hierarchy of consultation, appropriate degrees of involvement/consultation will vary according to the particular project and the needs and capacities of the young people to be involved.

There are a number of common arguments provided in support of consulting with pupils. First, consulting with pupils not only identifies pupils' preferred and most effective way of learning but can also reveal insights into how to effectively provide opportunities that will strengthen their commitment to learning (Pollard et al., 1997). Secondly, developments in national Children's Acts highlight young people's moral, ethical and legal rights on being consulted on matters that affect them (United Nations Convention on the Rights of the Child, 1989; Davie and Galloway, 1996). Thirdly, as well as becoming more involved in the school community, consultation can help pupils develop life-skills such as communication, working collaboratively and articulating their thoughts and opinions (Rudduck and McIntyre, 2007).

How to Consult Pupils and What to Consult Pupils About

In what ways, and under what conditions, can the teacher realistically encourage and enhance pupils' engagement in being consulted? In what ways can the teacher respond to such consultations? A user-friendly pack entitled 'Hearing Young Voices' (McAuley and Brattman, 2003) provides guidelines for consulting children and young people while other references focus particularly on developing dialogue about teaching and learning (Macbeath et al., 2003; Flutter and Rudduck, 2004). For consultation to flourish and survive conditions in the classroom for developing consultation include trust, respect, recognition and time to reflect.

Pupils have been consulted about school-wide, year group and classroom issues. Teachers need to consider legitimate pupil concerns appreciating that teachers can learn from pupils about what and how to teach. The Consulting Pupils about Teaching and Learning Project includes six constituent projects that foreground pupils' perspectives about teaching and learning and the ways in which teachers can develop effective ways of enhancing pupil engagement (Rudduck and McIntyre, 2007).

Reflection: Considerations for Actively Involving Pupils in Discussions and Decisions

When considering involving pupils in discussions and decisions that are expected to result in identifying more effective learning opportunities you should consider the following (adapted from Alderson, 1995):

1. The purpose of the consultation
2. Have the pupils helped to identify and plan the explicit purpose of the consultation? If the consultation and subsequent findings are to benefit certain pupils, who are they and how might they benefit? Can the exclusion of pupils for particular reasons be justified? Do pupils know they can refuse or withdraw from their involvement at any time?

Costs and hoped-for benefits

Might there be risks or costs such as time, sense of failure or coercion, or embarrassment? Are the pupils made aware of possible benefits, risks and outcomes?

Privacy and confidentiality

Is it possible for pupils to remain anonymous when significant extracts from their discussions might best qualify the need to reconfigure learning opportunities?

Dissemination

Will the pupils be involved in disseminating the outcomes of discussions and decisions within the school and to their parents?

Caution in Consultation

The unprecedented international interest in pupil consultation has led some to warn that we not lose sight of grounding such an interest in worthwhile and defensible principles and practices (Rudduck and McIntyre, 2007). There is an assumption that the value of student voice to school improvement is often a good thing and it is important to be aware of occasions when consultation with young people is inappropriate or exploitative (McAuley and Brattman, 2003).

It is imperative that young people are afforded meaningful, equitable and sustainable opportunities to be heard. A tokenistic approach to consultation, where pupils' contributions are directed and structured by the teachers' agenda, is worse than not consulting at all and will be counterproductive. It is also important to classify what 'consultation' means, what can and cannot be expected of involvement in a consultation and whether or not pupils have a preference for facilitation by someone they know (McAuley and Brattman, 2003).

Feeding back to pupils following consultation is essential and involves sharing the findings and informing pupils on how their contributions have informed decisions and actions. Asking young people to evaluate the consultative process in which they have been involved is vital to improving future interactions. While there is an increasing wealth of information on what schooling means in the lives of young people and what pupils say about issues related to teaching and learning, there is little published research exploring and reporting what pupils' perspectives are on being involved in consultation practices (Rudduck and McIntyre, 2007). Morgan (2008) examines pupils' understandings of consultation in general and their perspectives on all classroom consultation that takes place. While pupils reported welcoming consultation, having much to say about the benefits of consultation for their learning and their teachers' teaching, they were conscious of issues of trust, anonymity and not upsetting teachers. Pupils felt that not all teachers could be trusted to the same extent, were concerned that information gained from consultation could be used against them and did not want to offend teachers because of the possible consequences for themselves as well as a genuine concern for teachers.

Pupil Consultation Specific to Physical Education

The 2005 monograph of the *Journal of Teaching in Physical Education* (Graham, 2005) presents the findings of studies that specifically investigated the way pupils experienced elementary/primary physical education. In his review of pupil perspectives Dyson (2006) reports on pupils' views, experiences and perspectives of physical education, focusing on the physical education curriculum, pupils' likes and dislikes in physical education and pupils' perspectives of innovative curriculum. Drawing from these two sources, the compiled studies indicate that pupils (1) inherently enjoy being active in interesting and fun activities, (2) enjoy taking part in some form of (competitive) game play, (3) would appreciate a wider variety of activities and more input into their activity choices, (4) have a preference for particular activities, (5) enjoy the social aspect of being involved in physical activity, (6) appreciate learning activities that allow them to achieve a sense of success, (7) at times feel alienated from learning experiences that are not enjoyable, interesting or motivating, and (8) report that showering and changing can be barriers to participation. Variables that have been identified as influencing pupils' thoughts on physical education include age and gender, beliefs about their own ability and competence, beliefs about the value of a task and goal orientation.

While there is acknowledgement that pupil consultation is an important aspect in designing a relevant physical education for young people, there is little referenced work on how such values and beliefs have informed the development of effective practice in physical education (Brooker and Macdonald, 1999; Ennis and McCauley, 2002) or how pupil voice can contribute to the construction of what Glasby and Macdonald (2004) term a 'negotiated curriculum', curriculum designed in partnership with teachers. Rikard and Banville (2006) support teachers soliciting and considering pupil voice in physical education curriculum modifications that are educationally appropriate and that increase participation and motivation.

One innovative study developed a new physical education unit that was pupil-directed and examined curriculum negotiation in physical education (McMahon, 2007). The focus was on one class of 10–11 year old Irish pupils' views of their involvement in curriculum negotiation and how it affected their investment and ownership of the physical education curriculum. The researcher acted as the teacher and the study was undertaken in two parts. Phase one involved pupils' participation in a Sport Education unit, designed to give them more responsibility for their learning through an increase in decision making from previous physical education classes. Following the recommendations made by pupils after phase one, phase two involved pupils in a process of curriculum negotiation with the researcher / teacher in which they determined the purpose, content, aims, teaching methods and assessment of the physical education curriculum. Numerous reasons were shared by pupils for claiming that this physical education experience was one of their best. These included 'the nature of the activity being dance (something the students rarely got to do), student learning that was consistent with objectives students created, students feeling more involved in the lesson, and students having greater responsibility and getting to make decisions' (McMahon, 2007, pp. 92–93). In this project, pupils were not simply involved as subjects in the collection of data but had agency in defining, extending and providing direction for the physical education curriculum collaboratively with the researcher/teacher. This encouraged pupils to identify those issues that they (and not necessarily the researcher/teacher) felt were of importance in their experience of physical education.

Seeking 'voice' from particular populations involved in physical education and sport are sought and these include adolescent girls (Oliver and Lalik, 2001), young disabled people (Fitzgerald, 2005) and disengaged youth (Sandford et al., 2008). However, Groves and Law (2003) warn researchers/teachers to be cognizant of not treating members of a specific population as one entity but rather acknowledge that there are cultural and social vagaries that constitute individuals even within an identified population. This is another challenge to eliciting pupils' voice.

Traditional methods of seeking pupils' perspectives, such as questionnaires and interviews, often restrict and prescribe content for discussion with pupils' voice subsequently limited to opinion on specific issues pinpointed by the researcher rather than the pupil (Groves and Law, 2003). While research interested in gaining a better understanding of children's motivational process and achievement behaviours has relied on models and theories (not necessarily acknowledging the social influences on young people in contemporary society) to explain motivational patterns, methodological considerations encouraging a level of sophistication in listening to, and positioning, student voice, as well as involving pupils in guiding the educational research process, are becoming more evident in physical education, and related, research. These include the use of narratives (Enright and O'Sullivan, 2007), drawings (MacPhail and Kinchin, 2004), diaries (Lines, 2007), magazine exploration (Oliver and Lalik, 2001), photography (Pope, 2007) and ethnographies (O'Donovan and Kirk, 2008). Discursive practice through which we examine how young people construct their identity (beliefs and values) and position themselves in relation to their school context and the larger sociocultural context outside the school extends and contextualizes teachers' understanding of pupils' reality (Sandford and Rich, 2006).

Reflection: Involving Students in Curriculum Design and Development

Pupil drawings and pupils working in small groups to construct a poster are ways in which teachers can be encouraged to avoid limiting pupils' voice to opinion on specific issues pinpointed by the teacher. By asking pupils to draw an image of their experience of school physical education, without any further prompts, and then encouraging them to explain their drawing to the teacher, teaching and learning issues pertinent to the current provision of physical education will arise. A follow-up activity would be to ask pupils to draw a second picture, this time denoting an image of what they would like their experience of school physical education to be. This will encourage a space for pupils to share their views with the teacher on how they would like the Physical Education curriculum to be constructed. Similarly, encouraging pupils to work in groups to construct a poster that illustrates the creation of a Physical Education curriculum based on their needs and interests has potential to involve students in curriculum decision-making. These posters can be shared with the class and discussion can ensue between the pupils and teacher on ways in which the pupils' contributions can inform a particular physical education unit of work.

In both instances, feeding back to the pupils is essential and involves consulting and sharing with them ways in which their contributions have informed resulting decisions and actions.

Extending Pupil Voice

A potential extension of the school-focused interest in listening to pupil voice is prompted by Vadeboncoeur (2006) who encourages engagement with young people's learning in informal contexts such as extra-curriculum programmes, community organizations, family and friendship groups. This offers a clear link to those of us involved in teaching physical education with an aim to motivate the pupil to choose a lifestyle that is active, healthy and meaningful. By encouraging young people to share how different contexts contribute to their learning about, and involvement in, physical activity we may be in a better position to acknowledge and address how physical education and such contexts can most effectively work together to motivate pupils to choose active lifestyles.

The traditional power dimension between the pupil and the teacher needs to be challenged to redefine the boundaries of possibility (Rudduck and Fielding, 2006). Recently, primary-aged pupils reported the pupil–teacher dyad as comparable to 'ants versus giants' where, in the context of school physical education experiences, pupils perceive teachers (the giants) as those who boss the student (the ants) around (McMahon, 2007). A mix of pre-conditions and commitment in a particular school that create a more collaborative teacher–pupil relationship, where learning is accepted as a joint responsibility, have been identified as having guidelines for policy-makers in schools that help to define the more specific conditions in which consultation can flourish (Rudduck, 2006). Pre-conditions include a classroom or school climate that is marked by trust and openness and encouraging teachers and pupils to see each other differently from traditional conceptions, believing that they can reciprocate with open and constructive dialogue about teaching and learning experiences.

> **Reflection**
>
> ## Assessment (and teaching) for learning
> Formative assessment is intended to enhance pupil learning through frequent opportunities to provide evidence of their understanding, which in turn will help individual pupil progress. Assessment for learning extends to informing pupils about their own learning, acknowledging that they are decision-makers in their own learning. One example would be to construct a report card for each unit of work in physical education, identify a number of related learning outcomes and allow a space for the Physical Education teacher and the pupil to denote the extent to which each believe the pupil achieved each outcome. As an outcome, the completed report cards could contribute to an annual pupil profile as a way, for pupils and teachers, to assess pupil development and progress. This not only serves the purpose of alerting parents to the pupils' progress but also acts as a facilitation tool in the pupil–teacher discussion on co-creating plans to continue and expand their learning.

While it seems that within physical education we have examined pupils' experiences and understandings of the physical education context there is a lack of evidence regarding the extent to which students' perspectives have impacted the practice and research of physical education (Dyson, 2006). Encouraging pupils to design and undertake their own research (a shift from what Fielding (2001) terms students as data sources or active respondents to co-researchers or researchers) is a promising way in which to hear the voices of pupils in areas that they identify and believe to be crucial to their sense of membership in the school as a learning community. Considering how to build capacity and help pupils as researchers become a more established feature of how the school operates is a further challenge.

Learning More

A number of sources have been written as a practitioner's introduction to considering the potential benefits and implications of consulting with pupils about teaching and learning (e.g. Fielding and Bragg, 2003; McAuley and Brattman, 2003; Rudduck and Flutter, 2003; Flutter and Rudduck, 2004). The assumption that young people are active participants in their own lives and that they are entitled to a voice in matters that affect them is evident in published reports concerned with well-being and recreation (e.g. Nic Gabhainn and Sixsmith, 2005; Office of the Minister for Children and Department of Health and Children, 2007).

References

Alderson, P. (1995) *Listening to Children: Children, Ethics and Social Research.* Barkingside: Barnados.

Booker, R. and Macdonald D. (1999) Did we hear you: Issues of student voice in a curriculum innovation, *Journal of Curriculum Studies*, 31(1), pp. 83–97.

Davie, R. and Galloway, D.M. (eds) (1996) *Listening to Children in Education.* London: Fulton.

Dyson, B. (2006) Students' perspectives of physical education (pp. 326–346). In D. Kirk, D. Macdonald and M. O'Sullivan (eds), *The Handbook of Physical Education*. London: Sage.

Ennis, C. and McCauley, T. (2002) Creating urban classroom communities worthy of trust, *Journal of Curriculum Studies*, 34(2), pp. 149–172.

Enright, E. and O'Sullivan, M. (2007) 'Can I do it in my pyjamas?' Negotiating a physical education curriculum with teenage girls. Paper presented at the British Educational Research Association Annual Student Conference, September, Institute of Education, London.

Fielding, M. (2001) Students as radical agents of change, *Journal of Educational Change*, 2(3), pp. 123–141.

Fielding, M. and Bragg, S. (2003) *Students as Researcher: Making a Difference*. Cambridge: Pearson.

Fitzgerald, H. (2005) Still feeling like a spare piece of luggage? Embodied experiences of (dis)ability in physical education and school sport, *Physical Education and Sport Pedagogy*, 10, pp. 41–59.

Flutter, J. and Rudduck, J. (2004) *Consulting Pupils: What's in It for Schools?* London: Routledge Falmer.

Glasby, T. and Macdonald, D. (2004) Negotiating the curriculum: challenging the social relationships in teaching (pp. 133–144). In J. Wright, D. Macdonald and L. Burrows (eds), *Critical Inquiry and Problem Solving in Physical Education*. London: Routledge.

Graham, G. (ed.) (2005) Physical education through students' eyes and in students' voices [Monograph], *Journal of Teaching in Physical Education*, 14(4).

Groves, S. and Laws, C. (2003) The use of narrative in accessing children's experiences of physical education, *European Journal of Physical Education*, 8, pp. 160–174.

Jackson, L. (2002) *Freaks, Geeks and Asperger Syndrome. A User Guide to Adolescence*. London: Jessica Kingsley.

Lee, A.M. (1997) Contributions of research on student thinking in physical education, *Journal of Teaching in Physical Education*, 16, pp. 262–277.

Lines, G. (2007) The impact of media sport events on the active participation of young people and some implications for physical education pedagogy, *Sport, Education and Society*, 12, pp. 317–334.

MacBeath, J., Demetriou, H., Rudduck, J. and Myers, K. (2003) *Consulting Pupils: A Toolkit for Teachers*. Harlow: Pearson Publishing.

MacPhail, A. and Kinchin, G. (2004) The use of drawings as an evaluative tool: students' experiences of sport education, *Physical Education and Sport Pedagogy*, 9, pp. 87–108.

McAuley, K. and Brattman, M. (2003) *Hearing Young Voices. Guidelines for Consulting Children and Young People in Relation to Developing Public Policy and Services in Ireland*. Dublin: Open Your Eyes to Child Poverty Initiative.

McMahon, E. (2007) 'You don't feel like ants and giants': Student involvement in negotiating the physical education curriculum. Unpublished Masters Thesis, University of Limerick.

Morgan, B. (2008) 'I think it's about the teacher feeding off our minds, instead of us learning off them, sort of like switching the process around': Pupils' perspectives on being consulted about classroom teaching and learning. Paper presented at the British Educational Research Association Annual Conference, September, Heriot-Watt University, Edinburgh.

Nic Gabhainn, S. and Sixsmith, J. (2005) *Children's Understanding of Well-Being*. Dublin: The National Children's Office.

O'Donovan, T. and Kirk, D. (2008) Reconceptualising student motivation in physical education: An examination of what resources are valued by pre-adolescent girls in contemporary society, *European Physical Education Review*, 14, pp. 71–91.

Office of the Minister for Children and Department of Health and Children (2007) *The Report of the Public Consultation for the Development of the National Recreation. Policy for Young People*. Dublin: The Stationery Office.

Oliver, K.L. and Lalik, R. (2001) The body as curriculum: learning with adolescent girls, *Journal of Curriculum Studies*, 33, pp. 303–333.

Pollard, A., Thiessen, D. and Filer, A. (1997) *Children and Their Curriculum: The Perspectives of Primary and Elementary School Children*. London: Falmer.

Pope, C. (2007) Sport pedagogy through a wide-angle lens. Paper presented at the 2007 History and Future Directions of Research on Teaching and Teacher Education in Physical Education Conference, October, Pittsburgh, Pennsylvania.

Rickard, G.L. and Banville, D. (2006) High school student attitudes about physical education, *Sport, Education and Society*, 11, pp. 385–400.

Rudduck, J. (2006) Editorial. The past, the papers and the project, *Educational Review*, 58, pp. 131–143.

Rudduck, J. and Fielding, M. (2006) Student voice and the perils of popularity, *Educational Review*, 58, pp. 219–231.

Rudduck, J. and Flutter, J. (2003) *How to improve your school: Giving pupils a voice*. London: Continuum.

Rudduck, J. and McIntyre, D. (2007) *Improving Learning through Consulting Pupils*. London: Routledge.

Sandford, R., Armour, K. and Warmington, P. (2006) Re-engaging disaffected youth through physical activity programmes, *British Educational Research Journal*, 32, pp. 251–271.

Sandford, R. and Rich, E. (2006) Learners and popular culture (pp. 275–291). In D. Kirk, D. Macdonald and M. O'Sullivan (eds), *The Handbook of Physical Education*. London: Sage.

Kushman, J. (1997) *Look Who's Talking Now: Student Views of Learning in Restructuring Schools*. Portland: Northwest Regional Educational Laboratory.

Treseder, P. (1997) *Empowering Children and Young People: Promoting Involvement in Decision Making*. London: Save the Children and Children's Rights Office.

Vadeboncoeur, J.A. (2006) Engaging young people: learning in informal contexts, *Review of Research in Education*, 30, pp. 239–278.

United Nations (1989) *Convention on the Rights of the Child*. Geneva: United Nations.

Useful Resources

Organizations

Teachers of physical education are well-advised to consider membership of their national professional association. Apart from a greater sense of community and shared interest, these groups usually offer insurance, advice and resources.

Association for Physical Education (UK) – http://www.afpe.org.uk/
American Alliance for Health, Physical Education, Recreation and Dance – http://www.aahperd.org
Australian Council for Health, Physical Education and Recreation – http://www.achper.org.au
Physical Education New Zealand – http://www.penz.org.nz
Physical and Health Education Canada – http://www.phecanada.ca/

There are many international groups with an interest in the promotion of high quality physical education. The 'big five' groups are:

the Association Internationale des Ecoles Supérieures d'Education Physique (AIESEP) – http://www.aiesep.ulg.ac.be
the Fédération Internationale d'Education Physique (FIEP) – http://www.fiep.net
the International Association of Physical Education and Sport for Girls and Women (IAPESGW) – http://www.iapesgw.org
the International Federation of Adapted Physical Activity (IFAPA) – http://www.ifapa.biz
the International Society for Comparative Physical Education and Sport (ISCPES) – http://www.iscpes.org

The easiest way to access information about international developments is via the international umbrella organization, the International Council of Sport Science and Physical Education (ICSSPE) – www.icsspe.org

Key Texts

There are a few reliable textbooks on good practice in teaching physical education, and therefore might supplement this book. Among the best are:

Bailey, R.P. (2001) *Teaching Physical Education – a Handbook for Primary & Secondary School Teachers*. London: Kogan Page.
Mawer, M. (1995) *The Effective Teaching of Physical Education*. London: Longman.
Rink, J. (2006) – Sixth edition. New York: McGraw-Hill.

Other useful books, that will extend the themes discussed in this book include:

Bailey, R.P. and Kirk, D. (eds) (2009) *The Routledge Reader of Physical Education*. London: RoutledgeFalmer.
Kirk, D., Macdonald, D. and O'Sullivan, M. (2006) *Handbook of Physical Education*. London: Sage.

The *Reader* is collection of classic and influential papers on the theory and practice of physical education, with useful guidance on further reading. The Handbook is made up of specially written chapters on key themes.

Key Journals

Reading journals is a great way of keeping up-to-date on research, and of feeling a part of the community of scholars working in physical education. The leading international research journals are listed here.

Sport, Education and Society (UK) – http://www.tandf.co.uk/journals/titles/13573322.asp
Physical Education and Sport Pedagogy (UK) –http://www.tandf.co.uk/journals/titles/17408989.asp
European Physical Education Review (UK) – http://epe.sagepub.com/
Journal of Teaching Physical Education (US) – http://www.humankinetics.com/JTPE
QUEST (US) – http://www.humankinetics.com/quest
AVANTE (Canada) – http://www.cahperd.ca/e/avante/index.htm
Healthy Lifestyles Journal (Australia) – http://www.achper.org.au/publishing.php?id=160434

Other useful sources of information are those published by professional associations for physical education, such as:

Physical Education Matters (UK) – http://www.afpe.org.uk/public/member_journals.htm
Journal of Physical Education, Recreation & Dance (US) – http://www.aahperd.org/aahperd/template.cfm?template=johperd_main.html
Physical and Health Education Journal (Canada) – http://www.phecanada.ca/eng/journal/index.cfm
Active & Healthy Magazine (Australia) – http://www.achper.org.au/publishing.php?id=160423

All the websites mentioned under 'Useful Resources' were last accessed on 27 September 2009.

Appendix A
An Educational Timeline and Autobiography

Educational Timeline

Your task is to develop an educational timeline that displays how you have come to your decision to become a Physical Education teacher. Identify important people or 'critical incidents' that significantly influenced your thinking about the aims of education, Physical Education, and physical activity, about the role of professionals in our field, and how you fit into that role (A 'critical incident' is an event that has a big impact on you and causes you to make a change in your thinking or your actions. It is an event that has a great deal of meaning for you and who you are).

Consider your experience in school and in sport, how these environments felt to you, how you best learned, how you were treated, and when you felt most valued, connected, and involved – or least valued, most disconnected, and most uncomfortable. Consider the friends, coaches, teachers, and family members that influenced your participation and ultimately your decision to become a physical educator.

Steps in Developing Your Educational-decision Timeline

Step 1: Develop a list of the people who have had a major impact on your life and on your decision to teach Physical Education.

Step 2: Identify those events or critical incidents that you believe caused you to make a major shift in your beliefs or behaviour or influenced your views on teaching Physical Education.

Step 3: Develop an educational lifeline that reflects the positive and negative influences of these people and critical incidents.

Step 4: Place the positive influences/incidents above the line and the negative below the line.

BIRTH ━━━━━━━━━━━━━━━━━━━━━━━━━━━━━━━━ PRESENT

Step 5: Display your educational lifeline professionally on a sheet of paper or chart using large lettering so that it can be seen easily from a distance. Be prepared to discuss it with your peers.

Educational Autobiography

Once you have completed your education timeline, use it to guide the writing of your life story and your decision to become a teacher. You will find that as you start to write this narrative the memories and their implications will become clearer. You should come away with a better sense of who you are and where you are going in relation to your chosen profession. The process of writing this life story will also provide you with a better sense of your beliefs and perceptions about the role of a teacher and a physical education teacher in today's schools.

Visual Enquiry

As you develop your autobiography you may wish to draw an image of the type of teacher you would like to be in your classroom. Let your image form naturally in your consciousness and be led by your pencil.

On drawing, take time now to explore the image. Reflect with the help of the following questions:

- Describe what you have drawn.
- Where have you positioned yourself in the classroom?
- Where have you positioned your pupils?
- What are you doing in the drawing?
- What are your pupils doing?
- How are you dressed?
- How is the room organized?
- What objects are in the classroom?
- What is the feeling emanating from this picture?
- Would you like to be a pupil in this classroom?
- How are you feeling as a teacher in this classroom?
- What other questions could you ask about your drawing?
- What questions do you have for your peers on their drawings?

By engaging with your text and asking *why* to these questions you will challenge yourself to 'see' (inner perception) beyond the lines and colour. It may also be interesting for you to apply Diamond's (1991) threefold guiding questions to your developing images as a teacher: 'What do my images tell me about (a) the teacher I am, (b) the teacher I would like to be, and (c) the teacher I fear becoming'? Of course dialoguing with your peers, tutors, lecturers, mentor teachers, and professors, will help you to use these visual texts to further develop your understandings of teaching.

Appendix B
Collage Work

Clare's Collage

The following is an example of a collage by Clare, a physical education student, who is representing her understanding of what it is to teach before her first teaching practice placement and then again after she has completed her placement. Read this collage and based on your interpretation of these images, what overall picture do they give you about Clare's teaching experience?

Before teaching practice

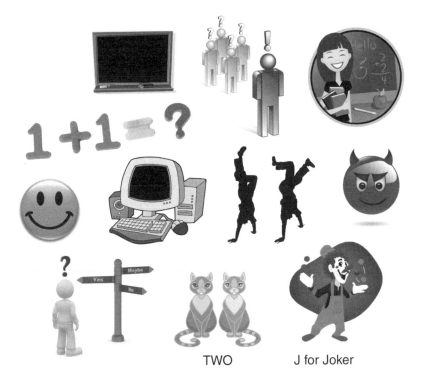

TWO   J for Joker

In reading this collage what do you think are Clare's understandings of teaching? How are they the same or different to your own understandings? If you were to track the development of your collage over time what might it look like? What are you adding or taking from your collage?

Teaching practice

During teaching practice placement Clare presented a set of images in her collage which included the following:

Week 1: Clare chose the painting, '*The Scream*' by Edward Munch to express her feelings about the first week of teaching practice. She writes:

> I chose this image to illustrate that I am lost at the moment and I feel like a traveller entering the unknown and frightening lands.

Week 6: In her final week of teaching practice Clare chose an image of a peacock. She writes:

> This may seem strange to you but if you look closely it represents a peacock. The proud peacock expresses how I felt in the last week of teaching practice. The students connected the learning and the discrete strands came together in an overwhelming whole of understanding.

Reflection

Can you identify with any of these images following your teaching practice?
What images would you choose and why?
Dialogue about these images with peers and faculty.
What more have you learnt from this dialogue?
Add your new learning to your existing images.

Appendix C
Guided Peer Reviews of Teaching

Teacher Observation

This guided observation focuses on the teacher, how the teacher explained the lesson and tasks to be learned, and managed the classroom.

> Observe your teaching peer as he/she completes their teaching focusing on the behaviour of the teacher not the students. Look for evidence and respond to the following prompts:
>
> > Comment on how well the teacher explained the lesson objectives/focus to the students. What evidence suggested students understood what they were going to learn in this lesson?
> >
> > Comment on the clarity of skill and practice task explanations and demonstrations the teacher gave to students. Could you understand what to do and how to do it?
> >
> > Comment on the teacher's enthusiasm and overall interaction with learners.
> >
> > Comment on how well the teacher managed the classroom using quick and efficient transitions and active supervision.

Learner Observation

This guided observation focuses the students, how they engaged and what they learned in this lesson.

> Observe the learners during your peer's teaching lesson today focusing on the learners not the teacher. Look for evidence and respond to the following prompts:
>
> > Comment on how well the learners knew what to do and where to go.
> >
> > Comment on how engaged (on task) the learners were during the lesson (or you can pick a specific aspect of the lesson).
> >
> > Comment on what you think the learners learned today. What evidence do you have for this learning? Were there different types of learning?
> >
> > Comment on if and how well the learners enjoyed the lesson. What evidence do you have for this?
> >
> > Were there some students who appeared to be more engaged with this lesson than others? What evidence do you have for this? Why do you think this might be so?

Appendix D
Community Mapping

The purpose of this assignment is to help you gain a better understanding of the community where your teaching practice school is situated. In particular it is about gaining insight about the sport, recreation, and leisure infrastructure in the community and how you might link your lessons to opportunities for engagement in sport and physical activity after school.

In this mapping activity, you will document the assets and issues of living in this community. You then reflect on this information about the community and to use this information to better connect your lessons to the lives of students you will teach in this setting.

'Mapping' the neighbourhood with a camera, making rubbings, taking photos, and interacting with the people in the neighbourhood should allow you to 'see' the community with fresh or new lenses. It should take about two hours to complete the mapping activity. You will map the local area, collecting information and talking to people.

During the Community Mapping you will learn more about:

- Organizations that exist in the community
- Geography and architecture of the community
- Different kinds of recreation, sport and leisure infrastructure in the community

To complete the mapping experience you will:

- Explore a section of the community
- Gather artefacts and photos
- Present a map and collage of the community.

The report on your community mapping can consider some of these questions.

What did you find:

Interesting about the process?
Helpful about the process?
Difficult about the process?
Enjoyable about the process?

Which of the activities engaged you the most? Why?
How does this process and information relate to connecting learning in students' life contexts?
How could community mapping be useful in teaching your Physical Education classes?
What did you learn about the community that you did not know before?
What issues related to the community emerged from your mapping?
How would you apply this experience to Physical Education content and to working with students?
In what ways, if any, were your perceptions of the students/community changed or enhanced by this experience?

Appendix E
Student Shadow

The purpose of the student shadow is to allow you to begin to understand how students experience and make sense of their life in school. With the help of your co-operating teacher, identify two students and obtain permission to follow them for an entire school day. Pick students you find interesting and with different backgrounds from your own. Take notes that will help you to recall significant events or comments during the day. Do your best to get to know the students and understand his or her feelings about school.

The following questions are not designed to limit you if there is something additional that you are interested in finding out about the students and their experiences.

How does the student spend his/her day?
How much of the students' experience of schooling was like your own? What was different from your experience?

What seems most important to the student during the day?
What topics and issues demand attention?
What events were found upsetting or irritating?
What were the sources of his/her greatest pleasure and disappointment during the day?
How did teachers and other students respond to the students?

Who holds the power within the school?
How were the students' voices heard in shaping their educational experience?
How was teacher and administrator power experienced?
How did the students respond to their power, or lack of power throughout the school day?
What does this mean to you as a teacher?
How will the information you gleaned impact your beliefs, values, and philosophies about teaching Physical Education?

Appendix F
A Teaching Portfolio Assignment: Documented Evidence Portfolio

Throughout your teacher preparation programme you have demonstrated knowledge, skills, and dispositions through projects, exams and teaching performance. In these instances, the professors/lecturers selected how you would demonstrate achievement. The portfolio assignment is intended for you to document your professional growth and mastery through a selection of artefacts that you believe document your achievement. Reflect on your view of the key skills, knowledge, dispositions and characteristics of an effective teacher and determine what evidence you might use (e.g. assignments, instructional materials, reflective journals, pupil evidence of learning) to demonstrate achievement of each aspect you identified as critical. Make your choices wisely and ensure that you adequately portray your achievement of becoming an effective teacher throughout your entire teacher education.

Your Documented Evidence Portfolio will use a narrative type format including (1) a description and a copy of your performance evidence, (2) your interpretation of the relationship of the evidence to key aspects of teaching, and (3) an explanation of your understanding of how your evidence reflects what is known about 'good' teaching practice. Remember to include a copy of the evidence itself.

Assessment of the portfolio will focus on the narrative that accompanies each piece of evidence and how well you linked it to your understanding of best practice. In other words, documentation of the evidence is thorough, detailed, and specific demonstrating substantive evidence of knowledge, understanding and application. As you move through your teaching career you will find it helpful to maintain your portfolio continually documenting evidence of your professional development as a teacher and its impact on student learning.

Appendix G
Real-world Case Studies

The multi-ability approach discussed in this Chapter 16 is now the nationally accepted framework for developing talented students in PE in England and various CPD delivery and resource development has been used in its implementation (Youth Sport Trust, 2009). The following case studies exemplify the ways in which schools have adopted the multi-ability framework within their own Physical Education environments and allow for reflection in terms of their wider use. All of the resources mentioned within these case studies are available on the Youth Sport Trust website (www.gifted.youthsporttrust.org.uk).

Case Study 1

Teacher: Alex Nicholls, Head of Physical Education

School: The Long Eaton School, Nottingham

Case study title: Meeting the challenge of identifying and providing for talented young people in Physical Education.

What we wanted to do?

The initial aim was to review the way in which we identify and provide for talented young people in school. The department's starting point was triggered when we were asked to update a school based register of gifted and talented students across the school. An informal discussion ensued about how we recognize talent in Physical Education. At that moment it was recognized that we needed to have some common values and criteria to effectively identify talented pupils in Physical Education.

What we did?

Stage 1

The Head of department had an informal discussion with the other Physical Education departmental leaders from the schools within the local area. It was clear that schools worked in isolation and had a whole raft of policies, values and standards that were being applied inconsistently. The department also had concerns about their feeder schools and the lack of information that was made available about students joining the secondary school at the beginning of each academic year.

Stage 2

It was clear at this stage that the school needed support from colleagues within the School Sport Partnership (SSP). The Head of Physical Education contacted our SSP Partnership Development Manager (PDM) and the issues were explored. As a result we hosted a conference for the SSP headed by a specialist talent development consultant and all people who deliver or influence Physical Education within the area were invited. The conference was a huge success and brought talent identification and provision into the spotlight. People were able to share good practice and the work presented was received positively. It was considered refreshing that talent in Physical Education was not only to be based upon sports representation or performance.

Stage 3

A working group was set up to explore how we were going to implement the work from the conference and make an impact on gifted and talented students' experiences.

Stage 4

The new aims included:

- Develop a policy on Gifted and Talented Education that could be consistently applied across the area.
- Produce a list of Gifted and Talented pupils within the SSP.
- Provide for these pupils in the following ways:

  1. Create a performance programme across the community of schools. Pupils given a range of experiences based on performance. Sport specific specialists from the local schools to deliver a range of opportunities based on performance.
  2. Local Clubs to be invited to offer short taster sessions with these pupils. A range of sports is essential.
  3. Other talented groups to be formed based on the multi-ability model.
  4. A range of roles and responsibilities within sport to be provided for these students.
  5. A festival of talent in the area to be organized by the students identified.
  6. Students to be encouraged to use their skills to help deliver high quality Physical Education within the feeder primary schools.

Stage 5

The Big Picture: 'How the talent conference has influenced the delivery of Physical Education'.

The working party has reviewed case studies from other schools and has decided to use the multi-ability approach to develop the delivery of Physical Education in the following ways:

- The Long Eaton School are going to pilot the multi-ability approach into their new schemes of work relating to the KS3 'count me in' programme used as part of the new Key Stage 3 curriculum.

- The department are aiming to promote independent learning from their students with self-assessment materials.
- Members of the Physical Education department to explore pathways in sport other than performance.
- Pupils will be recognized for their contributions in ways other than performance.
- The approach towards recognizing skills and identifying talent is to be extended across the Performing arts faculty area.

Case Study 2

Teacher: Steph McCoy, Co-ordinator for Physical Education and Sport
School: Handsworth Grange Community Sports College
Title: Using Multi-abilities in Sport Education (MASE) to develop talented young people

What we wanted to do:

- Create a teaching and learning environment where young people could develop their abilities through athletics.
- Engage a group who showed poor organization skills and challenging behaviour.
- Develop self-esteem by delivering tasks that would acknowledge a wide range of abilities demonstrated by young people.
- Raise enjoyment and attainment of the group.
- Assess the suitability of MASE as a tool to identify talented performers, and to help develop those abilities that are considered essential for an elite athlete to succeed.
- Establish whether Multi-Abilities in Sport Education (MASE) using Multi-abilities could provide a vehicle to deliver the needs of the new National Curriculum 2008.

What we did:

- Delivered ten lessons of athletics through the vehicle of MASE.
- Structured the unit around a 'Mini Olympics' competition, dividing the group into three teams of equal ability (equal in terms of perceived cognitive, creative, social, physical and personal ability).
- Shifted responsibility from teacher to pupil to empower the pupils. They were responsible for: managing and leading their team; planning and leading their team warm up; collecting/looking after equipment; ensuring Physical Education kit was correct; measuring/recording events; judging/being officials; coaching and improving technique; designing practices to develop their technique; developing tactics.
- Delivered tasks where pupils were given every opportunity to develop the five abilities (cognitive, creative, personal, social and physical).
- Developed a points system to reward teams/individuals for everything from correct kit, attendance and teamwork to excellent organization, showing initiative and performing to a high standard. Weekly scores were promoted around school to raise the profile of the work.
- Awarded a gold medal to the winning team (the team with the most points after ten weeks), and certificates for silver and bronze positions.

The Difference It Made:

- Actively engaged all pupils in at least one of the roles that MASE offered, allowing them to flourish in that area.
- Increased self-esteem and enjoyment – pupils felt that their role in each event was valued. Emphasis was placed on the importance of all roles (e.g. team manager), not just their physical performance.
- Organization (e.g. bringing correct kit), attendance and effort levels improved. Any excused on health grounds pupils brought kit and effectively worked in a different role, enabling all to be involved and engaged in the learning process/competition.
- Behaviour of the group improved.
- Teamwork skills and leadership qualities were especially enhanced.
- Pupils' physical competence and confidence improved on all levels.
- Pupils became more aware of their strengths and areas for development in terms of the five abilities.
- Increased the number of opportunities to assess pupils (from a personal point of view I was able to take a step back at different stages to assess, as well as allowing pupils to be creative and flourish).
- Brought a determined, fresh and exciting ethos to the classroom from both a pupil and teacher perspective.
- Delivered tasks that were designed to stimulate pupils and develop their abilities, whatever level they were starting from.
- Successfully used MASE as a platform for Assessment for Learning and opportunities for peer/self assessment.
- Discovered that Sport Education provided a suitable vehicle to identify talented performers; those pupils who were already at a high level of physical performance were able to flourish in the other ability areas.
- Gave staff the tools to create and develop MASE in other Physical Education units of work across KS3 & KS4 to help deliver National Curriculum 2008.
- Helped the Sport Specialism impact on the wider school – with support from Physical Education, MASE has been adopted initially by the Science and Maths departments to help engage pupils and deliver National Curriculum 2008.

It Worked Because:

- Tasks within the unit of work were challenging and engaging, providing pupils with every possible opportunity to discover their special ability and to shine.
- The competitive element captured pupils' imagination and rewarded reliability, teamwork and excellence in each ability.
- Young people had ownership of their team by choosing their own name, logo, motto and team chant.
- Working as part of a team gave pupils a sense of commitment and solidarity.
- Each pupil's ability was acknowledged; they felt valued, regardless of physical ability. Even the most talented sports performers were engaged by being able to focus on developing other abilities such as creativity.
- Pupils thrived on the responsibility they were given in different roles.

- Teams were equal in ability: each week the scores were close ensuring all pupils felt they had a chance of winning the competition.

Case Study 3

Teacher: Ben Mallinson, Physical Education teacher
School: Westborough High School
Title: Creativity in Physical Education

We wanted to:

- Produce an assessment template that considers different ways in which young people may demonstrate creativity in Physical Education as part of a Multi-ability Profiling system
- Plan activities that provide opportunities for young people to reveal creativity in Physical Education lessons
- Apply a creativity assessment template during Physical Education lessons
- Develop the creativity of all young people through innovative games activities as a trial to inform development opportunities within the new Key Stage 3 curriculum
- Recognize high levels of creativity to inform the identification of Gifted and Talented pupils

Meeting the Challenge

What we did:

Working closely with a talent development consultant, we developed a user-friendly resource that could be applied to a range of games activities within curricular time. To support the identification of creativity, the resource featured an assessment template to enable the teacher to recognize different levels of creativity demonstrated by the young people as they performed different tasks.

Initially, tasks were structured to ensure all pupils had a common objective and starting point. However, the subsequent direction of the activities was often determined by the creative interpretation of the instructions and rules, promoting independent learning and development.

The difference this has made

As well as facilitating the identification of talented pupils, the activities also provided opportunities and a stimulus for all pupils to develop creative ability in Physical Education. The impact of identifying pupils across the range of multi-abilities has made a considerable difference to our department's outlook and the recognition of pupils' potential. As a Creative Arts and Business Enterprise, creativity and innovative learning is recognized and celebrated across the whole school. It is important that Physical Education also promotes and drives the values of our school ethos.

Why it worked?

The informed production of the initial resource was critical to the success of the project. For a busy department it was essential to implement a resource that could achieve an impact on our pupils learning in a relatively short space of time. Within a games scheme of work the variety and novelty of the activities within the creativity resource really helped to motivated and inspire the pupils to become engaged in the lessons.

Index

Page numbers in **bold** denote words that appear in figures.